Ending Back Pain

Ending Back Pain

5 Powerful Steps to Diagnose, Understand,
and Treat Your Ailing Back

JACK STERN, M.D., PH.D.

AVERY

a member of Penguin Group (USA)

New York

Published by the Penguin Group
Penguin Group (USA) LLC
375 Hudson Street
New York, New York 10014

USA • Canada • UK • Ireland • Australia
New Zealand • India • South Africa • China

penguin.com
A Penguin Random House Company

Most Avery books are available at special quantity discounts for bulk purchase for
sales promotions, premiums, fund-raising, and educational needs. Special books
or book excerpts also can be created to fit specific needs. For details, write:
Special.Markets@us.penguingroup.com.

Library of Congress Cataloging-in-Publication Data
Stern, Jack I.
Ending back pain : 5 powerful steps to diagnose, understand,
and treat your ailing back / Jack Stern, M.D., Ph.D.
          p.   cm.
Includes index.
ISBN 978-1-58333-546-8
1. Backache.   2. Backache—Treatment.   3. Self-care—Health.   I. Title.
RD771.B217S732   2014   2014004284
617.5'64—dc23

Printed in the United States of America
1   3   5   7   9   10   8   6   4   2

BOOK DESIGN BY TANYA MAIBORODA

To my wife, Judy,
whose wisdom guides my life

Illness is the most heeded of doctors: to goodness and
wisdom we only make promises; pain we obey.
—MARCEL PROUST

God whispers to us in our pleasures,
speaks to us in our conscience, but shouts in our pains:
It is His megaphone to rouse a deaf world.
—C. S. LEWIS

Contents

Preface

COULD CLAIM THAT IT was my wife's fault. The year was 1990, and over the Labor Day weekend we'd traveled to Martha's Vineyard to celebrate my birthday. Judy's gift to me was a "special" massage that she'd thoughtfully scheduled, with the idea that it would help ease my chronic low back pain. But this wasn't the usual massage rooted in the simple pleasures of Swedish wisdom. This was going to be an experience that had the masseuse gently walking all over my back. As I made myself comfortable on the cushioned table, I pictured a petite lady kneading my back muscles with her dainty feet. Instead, I met a rather robust, Teutonic-looking woman who proceeded to stomp across my back as I moaned and groaned in silence. I really didn't want to appear wimpy, but I finally had to stop the massage because the pain had taken hold of me and began to sear down my leg. I soon learned that all the narcotics on the island did little to interrupt the connection between my brain and my back pain.

If I had to describe the pain, I'd say that it felt like electrical shocks shooting down my right leg. Though it came on gradually, over several hours, I reached a point where I couldn't move or even find a comfortable position. I knew I was in trouble when the doctor in the ER offered to call the Steamship Authority and arrange for an emergency spot on the ferry to get me off the island. Luckily, we had taken our station wagon, so I had a reasonably comfortable ride home with the seat in the maximally reclined position. I never before appreciated Percocet and Valium so much!

Judy had called ahead to one of my colleagues, an anesthesiologist, who specialized in pain management so that by the time she dropped me off at the hospital, I had a team waiting to perform an MRI. Going by the images, they were prepared to perform a relatively quick and easy procedure. I had already diagnosed myself as having a disrupted lumbar facet joint, something you'll read about shortly. This procedure involved what's called a facet block, and I went home about an hour later, pain-free. I was fortunate to have such amazing access to proper medical care, and the knowledge to quickly figure out my problem. I know that millions of people are not as privileged when something goes so terribly wrong. This is in large part the reason why I wrote this book.

Without a doubt, that experience deepened my understanding of what many of my patients endure, and made me a more empathetic physician. It has allowed me to better understand their plight and have a profound appreciation for the mysterious and sometimes elusive nature of pain. It also has further empowered me to listen to and learn from them, for if I had to say what has influenced me the most throughout my career, it has been my patients. They have been my greatest teachers. Although we experience pain that is unique to each of us, there are patterns of pain—patterns that allow me to better understand the source of pain and enable me to venture a diagnosis and suggest a treatment plan based on how others with the same pattern found relief. In this respect, the diagnosis and treatment of back pain are no different from those for any other disease. They require a thorough history and physical exam; they also usually call for laboratory and/or imaging studies to confirm a diagnosis and identify a course of action that has been shown to be effective.

That said, what makes the treatment of back pain dramatically different from that of most other medical problems is of course the "pain" part. (For purposes of this book, "back pain," unless otherwise specified, will refer to low back pain. Wherever necessary, I'll refer to other types of back pain specifically.) My patients have also taught me that pain, especially if it goes undiagnosed or is improperly treated, frequently takes on psychological and social ramifications, all of which can change a person's life forever. To treat these individuals demands a hefty dose of empathy and honesty—the patience to listen, the compassion to care, and the rectitude to admit failure when things go wrong. To treat these patients also demands the "art" of medicine that comes with time and experience. And on occasion, doctors like me find themselves in that wretched position of having to distinguish (as best we can) between a patient who needs medication and one who seeks it for the wrong reasons. I have to tell the difference between individuals who somehow benefit from the pain—a phenomenon that people usually don't recognize in their own behavior—from those who don't. So, in some regards, my job entails a mix of physiology, biology, and psychology. Frankly, that's all part of what makes my job so intensely complex, challenging, and yet richly satisfying. In order for a physician like me to treat patients in pain, I need to look inward and examine all the moving parts aside from the pain.

A Method to the Madness

The statistics are sobering. Back pain is the second most common neurological ailment in the United States—only headaches are more common. And, after colds and influenza, it's the second most common reason Americans see their doctors. At some point, almost all of us will have an episode of severe low back pain that will adversely interfere with our quality of life. It's believed that low back pain costs the economy $50 billion to $100 billion annually. It's the most common cause of job-related disability, accounts for more than 149 *million* lost workdays per year in the United States alone, and is the third most common reason for emergency room visits.

That's a lot of sore backs. You'd think that if the vast majority of the population will experience back pain at some point, then there would be a national outcry for more relief. Despite remarkable advances and new and better ways to diagnose and treat back pain, the problem continues to grow at an alarming rate. Why? Back pain isn't simple, and the solutions aren't always straightforward. There is, however, hope. Looking at the problem as a person who both treats and has suffered from back pain, I believe I have an insight that others might not.

As a board-certified neurosurgeon specializing in spine neurosurgery and as cofounder of Spine Options, New York's first and only center committed to nonsurgical care of back and neck pain, I've been on the front lines of the war on back pain for more than three decades and have treated more than 10,000 patients. My professional credentials are as a neurosurgeon, but I am acutely aware that surgery benefits only a select few. As such, my approach from start to finish is substantively different from those of most others in my field, and entails a multidisciplinary, holistic perspective that emphasizes the importance of a correct diagnosis *prior* to embarking on any treatment. In 1996, when I cofounded one of the nation's first in-hospital holistic healing centers, I committed to the idea that people can get better without surgery or similarly invasive procedures. I am also a staunch advocate of the philosophy that "less is more."

My motivation to write this book is simple: I'm alarmed by watching and reading all the misinformation about how to treat back pain. Every month in the United States alone, more than 4 million people Google the term *back pain* in hopes of finding information on why they hurt and what they can do about it. But what people find online is chaos—scattered information that's confusing and inconsistent, and an overload of biased, self-serving advertising for various treatments. What's more, back pain gets short shrift from both doctors and the general medical community, which is probably why chiropractors deliver about half of all back care in the country. And books or programs aimed to help back pain sufferers just don't do the issue justice. Either they present back pain as an illegitimate, suspect medical issue or they espouse a particular treatment regimen and don't address the multiple causes and potential remedies for back pain. Many spine-care professionals are familiar with just a limited menu of options and are unable to provide sound advice across the entire field. This has the unfortunate effect of leaving patients confused about which course to take.

In 2013, the topic hit headlines when a new study out of Harvard Medical School revealed that the number of people who have been prescribed powerful painkillers or referred for surgery and other specialty care have increased in recent years—despite guidelines to treat back pain conservatively. "Conservative management" in most cases means using aspirin or acetaminophen (Tylenol) and physical therapy during a wait-and-see approach rather than going directly to advanced imaging procedures, narcotics, and referral to specialists. In the study published in *JAMA Internal Medicine*, researchers looked at 23,918 outpatient visits for back pain, which was intended to reflect a sample of an estimated 440 million visits made over twelve years in the United States. After factoring out certain variables such as age, gender, and the nature of the pain, they found that during this time, over-the-counter, non-steroidal anti-inflammatory drug use (e.g., Aleve and Tylenol) fell 50 percent, while use of prescription opiates increased by 51 percent and CT or MRI scan tests rose by 57 percent. Meanwhile, referrals to other doctors climbed by 106 percent; the authors of the study pointed out that this likely contributed to the surge in expensive and often unnecessary spine surgeries.

This is alarming, to say the least. Although there is a time and place for painkillers and surgery, as this book will explain, few people are aware that there are safer, much more effective alternatives that can ease or eradicate back pain. Some of the strongest evidence, for instance, actually supports treating pain with exercise for certain types of back pain. And some 95 percent of people will recover from back pain without invasive or risky treatments. I find it telling that a

2012 Japanese study revealed that when adults suffering from chronic back pain visited an amusement park, they reported that their pain decreased significantly. But it came back once the trip was over. So much about back pain can be rooted in one's psyche and mind, a hotly contested subject matter that will be covered in this book.

Given the fact that most people will develop an aching back at some point, it shouldn't be viewed as an abnormal condition that necessitates costly medical care. We can probably change the entire back pain industry by just seeing it in a different light. Rather than approaching back pain as if it were an illness or disease, we should acknowledge it as a normal, inevitable aspect to aging that is for the most part ideally managed through patience and a change in lifestyle. Although most of us prefer quick fixes, sometimes the best advice is to wait and see.

Simon Dagenais, D.C., Ph.D., a prolific researcher who conducts studies to support evidence-based management of spinal and orthopedic disorders, articulated it perfectly when he said that choosing a treatment for back pain is akin to "shopping in a foreign supermarket with illegible product labels when one is hungry." Indeed, there are hundreds if not thousands of possible treatments for back pain, plus dozens of diagnostic approaches. The question is, though, how does the average person navigate all the options and know which is best? And how can a patient learn to be an advocate for his or her health without worrying about being a difficult patient? This book will help you answer these perplexing questions to get the back pain relief you need that is most appropriate for your condition.

A Little History

Lower back pain has afflicted humans for as long as we've roamed the planet. It's an experience nearly as universal as the common cold. In 2003, Drs. Guido R. Zanni and Jeannette Y. Wick wrote a marvelous, well-documented piece for the *Journal of the American Pharmacists*

Association titled "Low Back Pain: Eliminating Myths and Elucidating Realities." In it, they chronicle the history of back pain from ancient times to the modern era, describing early evidence dating back to an Egyptian papyrus from 1500 BC that may be the first written clinical description, and suggests the treatment of lying down. Biblical references to back pain include the famous one in Genesis in which Jacob is suffering from sciatica after he struggles with an angel. During the Middle Ages, people turned to folk medicine for help with their pain because they believed that supernatural causes created such discomfort.

Formal writings on back pain didn't really emerge until the 1800s, when physicians finally began to connect back pain with trauma or injury. Up to that point in time, most doctors believed the pain was a form of rheumatism or lumbago, which refers to pain in the muscles and joints. But even then, as today, visible pathology didn't necessarily translate to predictable symptoms that made sense. One can have clear evidence of damage on an imaging test, for instance, but have absolutely no pain—or vice versa, whereby there's pain but no obvious source for the pain seen on an X-ray, CT scan, or MRI, or with other imaging technology.

Although doctors didn't have a handle on back pain throughout much of history, surgery to alleviate the pain has long been among the most common, and most invasive, of medical procedures. One can only imagine the kind of primitive forms of medical treatments that were applied to back pain patients who were desperate to end their misery. In the fifteenth century, the surgeon Şerefeddin Sabuncuoğlu detailed lower back pain in handwritten manuscripts with illustrations. His recommendations for treatment included the use of analgesic medications and, when warranted, a cauterization (burning) procedure.

Dr. Sabuncuoğlu was right to prescribe analgesics to help back pain originating from trauma or injury. Even his surgical interventions may have been helpful for stubborn pain if he managed to hit the exact area from where the problem emanated. After all, how different is this from the common practice of trigger-point injections, a type of pain treatment by which areas of muscular pain are injected with anesthetics and steroids to alleviate the pain? Modern options for treating back pain go back hundreds of years as well. Today's inversion tables and matted platforms consisting of pulleys, ropes, and weights to relieve back pain are reminiscent of contraptions from the Middle Ages. By some standards, they may look like tools for torture.

Zanni and Wick relate the events of the early twentieth century beautifully: ". . . as societies struggled to develop social systems to address worker disability, physicians and politicians debated the reality of back pain. Some called it a 'litigation symptom,' and eminent psychiatrists of the day, including Sigmund Freud and Pierre Janet, went so far as to label back pain as a pathologic manifestation of unconscious conflict. Back pain gained a reputation as an emotional, rather than real, affliction."

It was during this time period that health statisticians began tracking the incidence of lower back pain. By the 1950s, other areas of medicine, chiefly those that were revolutionized by antibiotics and insulin, grew by leaps and bounds. Vaccines changed the course of ailments such as polio and smallpox, and improvements in people's general lifestyle (i.e., diet and exercise) helped prolong our lives further, allowing us to live well into our seventies and eighties. But when it came to back pain, the pain persisted. What's more, an increasing number of workers' compensation claims brought back pain to the forefront of analysis.

Although it's now generally acknowledged that lower back pain is a serious and real medical problem, many people still choose to believe and give credence to biases of malingering. It's often considered a workers' compensation nightmare because costs of back pain claims are exorbitant, and it's undeniable that some workers do exploit or abuse the system. Experience, however, has shown me that few individuals are wildly exaggerating or faking their pain. In some patients there are disconnects between their symptoms and the findings on physical examinations and imaging studies. In other words, someone whose symptoms don't match a valid diagnosis or pathology is often suspected of "symptom magnification." I also believe that almost all patients who demonstrate this disconnect are unaware of their behavior, a phenomenon I'll explore.

With this book I hope to present a new paradigm for the diagnosis and treatment of back pain. You may not find your personal solution on the very first page (or maybe you will), but my goal in this book is to equip every back pain sufferer with the information and power to get to the bottom of his or her own problem. In a world of rapidly changing technology, competing information, and an increasingly troubled health care industry, it may seem impossible to know what you need and, more important, how to get it. *Ending Back Pain* is your step-by-step companion to sleuthing your way to a more pain-free existence. Indeed, after centuries of searching for answers to this most common ailment, the time has come to put an end to the misery. As I hope to show in this book, the power to end back pain is within all of us.

Introduction

PERHAPS YOU'RE READING THIS while trying your best to avoid the next unbearable sensation of pain in your back. Maybe you've been dealing with back pain for a long time and are fed up with the ongoing, endless struggle for which you don't have a clear diagnosis or solution (or the original diagnosis and treatment didn't bring total relief). Or perhaps you're someone who has just begun to experience back pain and you're terrified that it will get worse over time, especially since your doctor has as yet been unable to pinpoint a real cause, much less a suggested cure. You don't know where else to turn, and you keep asking, *Why me? Will this come to define the rest of my life? What should I do now? How can I end the pain and prevent this from happening again?* The fear of living with chronic back pain looms large.

Regardless of your unique story and circumstances, I'm here to help you discover how to take charge of your back pain, and carry you to a place where you can live the most pain-free life possible. In five steps, you'll learn how to:

1. Unlock your back's unique code through an appreciation of the six major anatomical sites that can cause low back pain, which are called the pain generators, as well as non-anatomical causes of low back pain, such as drugs and underlying medical conditions or diseases. Put simply, Step 1 gives you a clear road map to use for getting to the bottom of your back pain's origins.

2. Be an advocate for yourself with health professionals. Step 2 supplies you with all the instructions and self-evaluations you need to then approach a doctor and optimize that relationship.

3. Ensure proper diagnosis. In Step 3, you'll learn in detail the whys and hows of pain emanating from the back's main pain generators, which will ultimately help you to get diagnosed correctly. You'll also get inside my head as I share what a doctor like me thinks when someone with your type of pain enters my office. Between the lessons learned and questionnaires you complete in Step 1, you'll have a much better idea about which type of pain is relevant to you so that you can make the most of Step 3.

4. Embark on a plan of treatment and recovery based on your individual diagnosis, one that will entail a wide variety of options from least to most invasive. Step 4 reveals all the common approaches to back pain as well as offers a candid look at what happens when nothing seems to work—when the pain may actually come more from the mind than the back. Some of the solutions described in this step reiterate the treatments explained in Step 3, but the goal is the same: to help you make the most of your journey to a pain-free back, whether that involves an integration of therapies or a single remedy.

5. Take advantage of strategies to prevent future back pain and live as much a pain-free life as possible. Finally, Step 5 showcases the strategies for ending back pain for life—offering my hope that future back pain treatment will improve and that there is a lot we all can do today to prevent back pain in the future. In the conclusion, I'll help you see how all five steps come together, stressing once again that the cure for back pain is rarely a magic bullet. It's an ongoing plan of action.

Although I've created a five-step program, this book does things a little differently. You'll find that there will be lots of crossover among the steps; this subject matter requires us to touch upon many of these steps at the same time. The information about being your own advo-cate in front of health professionals, for example, will relate directly to both understanding your unique pain and getting the right diagnosis. Similarly, your path to a pain-free back will demand that you respect your emotions and psychological circumstances while you consider specific anatomical problems that play into your back pain. In other words, healing your back pain involves an amalgamation of all five steps. I have organized this book to maximize your journey through these steps. And I'm going to start you off with a quick questionnaire, which will help you start gathering the clues you need to understand your own back, before leaping into Step 1.

Due to the volume of material covered, and to further help you to know exactly what to do, I've created itemized action plans wherever appropriate at the ends of certain chapters. They serve to both high-light key points and give you specific action steps to take, based on the information in that chapter. Some of these action steps may not be relevant to you, but you'll know how to distinguish between what's applicable to your type of pain and what's not. Virtually nothing about back pain is one-size-fits-all, so I've written this book to be user-friendly and adaptable to you, no matter what kind of back pain you're dealing with.

Of all the advice dispensed on alleviating low back pain, two over-whelmingly critical issues are frequently neglected. I will hammer these issues consistently throughout the book. One is diagnosis. End-ing back pain requires an accurate diagnosis, which many people do not receive. There are many reasons for this, and we'll be exploring how you can avoid this fate. And two, back pain is one of those few ailments that are manifested across a wild spectrum of the popula-tion. Put another way, no two back pain patients are exactly the same. Unfortunately, when most back pain patients talk to their doctors, the complaints fall on inattentive ears. Doctors hear about back pain so frequently that they've become desensitized to the problem, and in addition they know that most back pain resolves spontaneously without any interventions. As a result, they don't spend a lot of time thinking through solutions tailored to each patient's individual case. They typically offer a single remedy to all patients, which may not be the right one.

So, what happens when you have unresolved, persistent back pain? You are, quite honestly, a big problem for your doctor. How do I know this? Because that's how I felt before I began to think more critically about unrelenting back pain. Most physicians, when asked, won't hide their frustration about the prospect of dealing with back pain. It's a time-consuming, multifactorial quandary, which the average physician is not adequately trained to treat. It's the reason a whole new specialty of medicine was created in the 1990s, called pain management, and one I find myself practicing daily as a back pain doctor.

Before We Get Started

So, we begin our journey here with a few commitments that I ask you to make. By using this book, you are resolving to be your own advocate for getting the right diagnosis and care. I'll be sharing with you the knowledge you need to do this, but learning the information is only half the battle. You have to execute the lessons here. At the same time, open yourself up to understanding the main causes of back pain and the wealth of treatments available. I realize that some of you may think that as an active surgeon I will push surgical options. Far from it! The repertoire of potential treatments runs the gamut of choices, from traditional Western medicine to Eastern medicine to chiropractic and to integrative therapies such as Pilates and the Alexander Technique, to name a few. And if surgery is the ultimate recommendation, then this book will help you make that decision and be well informed about the pros and cons.

By and large, *Ending Back Pain* is intended to be the practical, hands-on guide that will help anyone with back pain find a more pain-free life—whatever that entails. For some of you, a "cure" could be having a totally pain-free back in just a few weeks using a certain protocol, or maybe it will mean that you feel better in a month and are able to function more easily at home or work but will still have some pain to manage. I know all too well that back pain tends to have more than one trigger, more than one source of agony. Your pain may not be caused by a well-defined diagnosis, such as a slipped disc. In fact, more frequently than not, the pain is rooted in a constellation of physical mishaps made all the more vexing by emotional, psychological underpinnings.

This is precisely why my "whole patient" approach to healing goes far beyond simply treating an ailing back. It's designed to get to the root of the problem of low back pain, even when the solution involves learning to live with some of the pain. Please use this book however you want to make the most of its information. As you read, highlight or circle anything about pain that seems relevant to you. Write in the margins or keep a journal to take notes and complete the exercises I'll be giving. To access the most up-to-date information and online tools that will help you take full advantage of the recommendations in this book, go to www.drjackstern.com. There, you'll be able to stay on top of the latest in back pain studies, learn about the most recent technologies that may be relevant to you, and view my ongoing blog and video content where I share what's going on in the back pain community.

By the end of this book, my hope is that you'll have gathered your own set of "symptoms," which is the first step to a diagnosis. I should point out that this book is not just for people who suffer from back pain, but it's also for your loved ones, who can help in the healing process. In addition to presenting the requisite "how to diagnose and treat" back pain, we're also going to explore some of the lesser-known facts related to the subject. For example, why is back pain practically nonexistent among certain populations? How much does the psychology of pain play into the biology of pain? And why will some patients never become pain-free regardless of proven solutions available to them? These questions, and so many more, will be answered. My ultimate goal is to inform and, of course, empower you to end your struggle with back pain. Back pain is not the enemy; our current way of addressing it is. It's time that you take control . . . and get your life *back*.

Step 1

Unlock Your Back's Unique Pain Code

IF I HAD TO SUM UP THIS ENTIRE BOOK IN A SINGLE PHRASE, IT would be this: Get to know your back. Ending back pain begins with you. One fact I'll be repeating over and over again is that diagnosing back pain is a tricky combination of art and science. Indeed, lots of high-tech tools are available to us in medicine, but that doesn't mean that diagnosing, let alone curing, back pain is a black-and-white endeavor. Unfortunately, it's very much to the contrary—complex, imprecise, and immensely vexing. So, the more you can contribute to the story of your back pain, the more you can shift your experience to one that's less reliant on art and more based on science.

As a prelude to Step 1, which will equip you with the information you need to decode your own unique pain, use the following checklist to organize your thoughts and personal information. This questionnaire is designed to help you prepare for a doctor's visit, giving you clues to what to discuss. But it should be filled out even before reading this book, because it will help you get to know yourself and your particular back pain better before embarking on this adventure. I also know that you want to be told what to do as soon as possible, and even though you'll find much to consider throughout this book, the following questions will provide you with concepts to think about as you read further and apply my ideas to your life. Your answers will help you get the most out of this book, and find a solution sooner rather than later.

The Checklist

Check off as many of the following questions that apply to you and bring this checklist with you to your doctor. Add additional notes where necessary.

This questionnaire is also downloadable online at www.drjackstern.com, where you'll find a version that you can fill out directly on the page, print for your records, and/or take to your doctor.

How long have you been experiencing back pain?
- ☐ within the past six weeks
- ☐ for more than six weeks

Do you have a personal or family history of any of the following:
- ☐ degenerative disc disease
- ☐ osteopenia or osteoporosis
- ☐ rheumatoid arthritis
- ☐ psoriatic arthritis
- ☐ urinary tract (bladder) infections
- ☐ kidney stones, urinary tract or kidney infections, or kidney disease
- ☐ any type of cancer (if so, which kind?)

Does your pain get worse by any of the following:
- ☐ engaging in a sport
- ☐ doing a certain activity
- ☐ sitting for a long period

- ☐ Is your pain relieved by rest?
- ☐ Is your pain relieved by non-steroidal anti-inflammatory drugs, such as Aleve (naproxen) and Advil (ibuprofen)?
- ☐ Does your pain radiate downward and stop somewhere? Where does it start? Where does it stop?
- ☐ Is your pain one-sided (on one side of your back or down one side of your leg)?
- ☐ Is the pain accompanied by a fever or weight loss?
- ☐ Does the pain occur when you stand, stretch, or sit?
- ☐ Is your pain worse in the morning and better at night?

☐ Is your pain better in the morning and more pronounced with activity?

☐ Does it intensify if you cough, sneeze, or move your bowels?

☐ Have you been injured or been in a recent accident?

☐ Have you recently participated in an activity or sport that you haven't performed in a long time (e.g., painting the house, raking leaves, playing dodgeball, exercising, skiing)?

☐ Do you have any soreness specific to a single muscle area, such as your hamstrings or quadriceps?

☐ Do you smoke?

☐ Are you overweight?

☐ Are you over the age of fifty-five?

☐ Do you have weakness in one leg that causes you to drag your foot?

☐ Do you experience tingling (a "pins and needles" sensation) or numbness in one arm?

☐ Do you have to turn your entire body to look over to the right or left?

☐ Do you feel pain in other areas, such as your shoulders, mid-back, buttocks, or thighs (but not below the knee)?

☐ Is it hard to stand up straight and get up out of a chair?

☐ Do you play tennis or golf?

☐ Was the onset of pain sudden and upon performing a specific act, such as bending to pick something up off the floor or reaching for a heavy box on a shelf?

How would you describe your pain?

☐ throbbing

☐ dull

☐ sharp

☐ burning

☐ shooting

☐ electrifying

☐ constant

☐ intermittent

☐ Does your pain serve you in any way? Are you addicted to your pain? Have you thought about what life would be like *without* the pain?

WHERE IS YOUR PAIN AND HOW DOES IT BEHAVE?

Draw your pain in the below figure. It can be a dot, a jagged line, a shaded section, and so on. If your pain travels from your back to somewhere in your front, make note of that in the margin and be as specific as you can. If you have a combination of issues, such as searing pain in one area and numbness in another, indicate that by using X's for the searing pain and Y's for the numbness. If the pain has changed over time, use more than one avatar and try to label it according to when the change occurred and if you know why.

Unlike other self-tests you may find in books and magazines, this one doesn't have a scorecard at the end. Your answers are your own. If you're

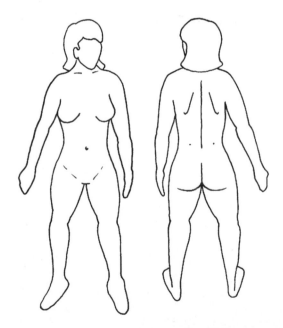

Where is your pain and how does it behave?

like most people, you may not even know what some of your answers mean, or exactly what to do with them. And that's okay. By the end of this book you'll know precisely how your responses will play into diagnosing and treating your pain. Once you've read further, and perhaps after applying some of my forthcoming suggestions, come back to this questionnaire to check in with yourself whenever you want. Or return to it when you think you can provide more comprehensive answers. If you weren't able to respond to one or more of the questions, you might be better equipped to do so once you've made more headway through the book. Mind you, there will be lots of opportunities to document your experience, as this book provides several self-tests and evaluations. But use this first checklist as your "cheat sheet"—your summary of main points related to your pain. Your responses could eventually turn into a game plan from which all treatment and preventive measures commence.

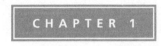

CHAPTER 1

The Science and
Art of Diagnosing Back Pain

M OST FEELINGS OF DISCOMFORT in life have clear solutions. For a stuffy nose, decongestants do the trick. For a pounding headache, aspirin or Tylenol comes in handy. But what do you do about a relentlessly aching back? As most of us know, the answer is not nearly as clear-cut as we'd wish. And unlike infectious diseases that often have targeted remedies (think antibiotics for bacterial infections and vaccines for viruses), ailing backs are like misbehaving, obnoxious family members—we can't easily get rid of them or "fix" them. They also have a tendency to stick around and bother us nonstop, lowering our quality of life considerably and indefinitely.

Perhaps nothing could be more frustrating than a sore or hurting back. It seems to throw off everything else in our body, and makes daily living downright miserable. With the lifetime prevalence approaching 100 percent, virtually all of us have been or will be affected

WHAT ARE THE CHANCES?

Chances are good that you'll experience back pain at some point in your life. Your lifetime risk is arguably close to 100 percent. And unfortunately, recurrence rates are appreciable. The chance of it recurring within one year of a first episode is estimated to be between 20 and 44 percent; within ten years, 80 percent of sufferers report back pain again. Lifetime recurrence is estimated to be 85 percent. Hence, the goal should be to alleviate symptoms and prevent future episodes.

by low back pain at some point. Luckily, most of us recover from a bout of back pain within a few weeks and don't experience another episode. But for some of us, the back gives us chronic problems. As many as 40 percent of people have a recurrence of back pain within six months.

At any given time, an astounding 15 to 30 percent of adults are experiencing back pain, and up to 80 percent of sufferers eventually seek medical attention. Sedentary people between the ages of forty-five and sixty are affected most, although I should point out that for people younger than forty-five, lower back pain is the most common cause for limiting one's activities. And here's the most frustrating fact of all: A specific diagnosis is often elusive; in many cases it's not possible to give a precise diagnosis, despite advanced imaging studies. In other words, we doctors cannot point to a specific place in your back's anatomy and say something along the lines of, "That's exactly where the problem is, and here's how we'll fix it." This is why the field of back pain has shifted from one in which we look solely for biomechanical approaches to treatment to one where we have to consider patients' attitudes and beliefs. We have to look at a dizzying array of factors, because back pain is best understood through multiple lenses, including biology, psychology, and even sociology.

The Challenge

So, why is back pain such a confounding problem? For one, it's lumped into one giant category, even though it entails a constellation of potential culprits. You may have back pain stemming from a skiing accident, whereas your neighbor experiences back pain as the consequence of an osteoporotic fracture. Clearly, the two types of back pain are different, yet we call them "back pain" on both accounts, regardless. Back pain has an indeterminate range of possible causes, and therefore multiple solutions and treatment options. There is no one-size-fits-all answer to this malady. That is why diagnosing back pain, particularly persistent or recurrent pain, is so challenging for physicians.

Some people are able to describe the exact moment or series of moments when they incurred the damage to their back—a car accident, a slip and fall, a difficult pregnancy, a heavy-lifting job at work, a sports-related injury, a marathon, and so on. But for many, the moment isn't so obvious, or what they *think* is causing them the back pain is far from accurate.

Before we begin to address your unique back pain, it helps to start with a grasp of the two main types of back pain and the three general types of patients.

The Two Types of Back Pain

If you are going to experience back pain, you'd prefer to have the acute and temporary kind rather than the chronic and enigmatic kind. The former is typically caused by a musculoskeletal issue that resolves itself in due time. This would be like pulling a muscle in your back during a climb up a steep hill on your bicycle or sustaining an injury when you fall from the stepladder in the garage. You feel pain for a few weeks and then it's silenced, hence the term *self-limiting* back pain. It strikes, you give it some time, it heals, and it's gone.

The second type of back pain, though, is often worse, because it's not easily attributed to a single event or accident. Often, either sufferers don't know what precipitated the attack, or they remember some small thing as the cause, such as bending from the waist to lift an object instead of squatting down (i.e., lifting with the legs) or stepping off a curb too abruptly. It can start out of nowhere and nag you endlessly. It can build slowly over time but lack a clear beginning. Your doctor scratches his head, trying to diagnose the source of the problem, and as a result your treatment options aren't always aligned with the root cause of the problem well enough to solve it forever. It should come as no surprise, then, that those with no definitive diagnosis reflect the most troubling cases for patients and doctors.

In addition to the two types of back pain, there are usually three types of patients. One is the person who has the right diagnosis but wrong treatment. Another is the individual with the wrong diagnosis and wrong treatment. And the third patient is the one you want to be: the one with the right diagnosis and the right treatment. My hope is that with this book you'll fill the shoes of this third patient. (As an aside, I should probably point out the potential fourth type of patient: the one with the wrong diagnosis but, miraculously, the right treatment. Though rare, this type of patient does exist. A correct diagnosis, however, is above all most important—especially if the pain returns and the treatment that worked initially is useless.)

The Cultural Factor

Does back pain discriminate? From a gender standpoint, back pain affects both sexes about equally (to be fair, back pain secondary to disc disorders is more common in men). But where it gets really interesting from a sociological perspective is the prevalence of back pain across different cultures.

It's no surprise that genetics can play a role in your lifetime risk for back pain. But what about your ethnicity? Your environment? The country in which you were born? Why do some cultures rarely experience back pain? Put another way: Is back pain "in your blood"? For a long time, the answers to these questions have intrigued researchers. As it turns out, where you are geographically affects what diseases you may have, even when it comes to back pain.

Perhaps the greatest demonstration of discrepancies among back pain sufferers can be found in comparing the two Germanys, once separated by the Berlin Wall. Between 1991 and 2003, researchers conducted five sequential health surveys to assess the prevalence of lower back pain among inhabitants of these two previously disconnected regions. What they discovered was quite astonishing: The first survey, done shortly after the reunification of the two countries, showed a much lower prevalence of lower back pain in East Germany compared to West Germany. But over the following years, up to 2003, the prevalence in the two countries became quite similar. How can this be? Such a shift cannot be attributed wholly to more accidents or trauma to people's backs. And it's doubtful that the East Germans suddenly experienced back pain like never before once they began commingling with their western counterparts.

The authors of this particular study, published in the *International Journal of Epidemiology*, hypothesized that the increase in back pain reported in East Germany was due to a "harmful influence of back-related beliefs and attitudes transmitted from West to East Germany via mass media and personal contacts." I would also surmise that with a united Germany there was now access to better health care and a social-service system that recognized and cared for workers who developed low back pain. In conjunction with that, what was probably happening is that people were changing their beliefs and attitudes about back pain and were giving themselves permission to talk about the subject. People went from hiding their pain to talking about it and being more aware of it. No longer would they just assume that back pain was a reality in life to silently endure. Now that back pain was being recognized in a way that it hadn't been previously, people were giving themselves permission to communicate their problem, complain about their pain, and seek help. Partly for this very reason, back pain is said to be "communicable."

The idea of back pain as a "communicable disease" is provocative. Certainly back pain is not a contagious illness like influenza or tuberculosis. But as more people talk about it and share their experience, more cases emerge, and it nonetheless entails a host of issues often attributed to "spreadable" or "infectious" ailments. Consider the following: We all are influenced by our social structures and how information gets disseminated. What we choose to complain about or act upon can easily be affected by the media or how our families train us to behave. Studies have also shown that different ethnic groups view pain and its expression differently. So, consider your own attitude about pain. As a child were you told to be a "big boy" or "big girl" and not be wimpy when you experienced pain? On the high school lacrosse team did you keep silent about the pain from your injury lest you be ridiculed or benched? Perhaps your parents were too preoccupied with their own issues and you learned to keep quiet when in pain. Or, conversely, you noticed that your brother's childhood illnesses got him the attention you craved, so you made sure to express your discomfort to get equal attention.

We can also be influenced by incentives. If a free back pain clinic opened up in our neighborhood, then we might find ourselves checking it out, and then we're accounted for as a back pain sufferer. Or, if we could gain monetary benefits by claiming to have back pain, then we might be inclined to do so when life gets rough. In Sweden, a country that differs from the United States in more ways than one, the level of insurance benefits for disabling low back pain is a breathtaking 100 percent, compared with the range of 0 to 80 percent here in the United States. In 1987, the percentage of the workforce placed on a sick list for a diagnosis associated with low back pain was 8 percent in Sweden versus 2 percent in the United States. In the same year, the average number of back-related absences from work per patient per year in Sweden was forty versus nine in the United States. Indeed, incentives can mean everything.

We must be careful, however, not to infer too much about the German study, because we actually lack sufficient information about the difference in prevalence of lower back pain in West and East Germany before the reunification. In light of the massive transformation of social structures in East Germany, many known and unknown variables (new political and economic systems, new health care and social-security systems) may have influenced the data sets. With more than 1.4 million people leaving East Germany in 1990, the population was not stable enough for researchers to make any inference about the reasons underlying the differences in back pain prevalence. Although the data were adjusted for age and gender, the researchers lacked specific information about other possible variables, such as socioeconomic factors, unemployment, risks such as physical workload, etc. It's also important to note that economic incentives or disincentives could have been involved, and certainly changes in the insurance system prior to reunification were influential as well.

Aside from the limitations to interpreting this data, the study is worth considering because it goes to show the complexity of the back pain problem. What's more, the inconsistencies found in Germany aren't unique to that region. Similar deviations have been found in other communities worldwide that further underscore the existence of compounding factors affecting the back pain story. Back pain, after all, can encompass a spectrum of ingredients across an even wider range of lifestyle components, from socioeconomic realities to personal ideologies and convictions.

Numerous psychological aspects may also be at play. That depression, anxiety, sleep disorders, and other neuropsychological conditions are often associated with chronic pain isn't news to most neurologists. But physicians who don't specialize in pain management are largely unaware of a growing body of research suggesting that a chronic-pain patient's race (a genetic classification) or ethnicity (a cultural classification) may determine his or her risk of neuropsychological symptoms.

In Step 4, I'll cover the role of the brain in the interpretation of pain signals and how the variety of these signals affects how you experience the pain—how the pain makes you "feel." You'll come to appreciate another side to pain's story and its biology. And within that story, we'll also find that one's cultural background and personal belief system can most definitely be an influential factor. Suffice it to say that researchers are beginning to piece together the race-pain puzzle, as evidenced by the increasing number of studies published in medical literature. Much of what investigators are learning, however, has yet to trickle down to the level of the treating physician.

This all brings me back to you: How much is your pain grounded in something—someplace—other than a specific spot in your back? That's the ultimate question I'm going to challenge you to ask and answer.

The Benefit of Being a "Spinal Generalist"

You may have encountered what I call the "back pain shuffle." That is what happens when your back pain does not go away and after several visits to your primary physician you are shuffled to a pain specialist, physical therapist, neurologist, chiropractor, orthopedist, or neurosurgeon.

According to a variation of the old adage, if you are a carpenter, the world looks like a bunch of nails to be hammered. So, what happens is the treatment you receive depends on the expertise of the specialist, the particular kind of carpenter you are sent to see. The physical therapist will start a rehabilitation program, the pain specialist may stick you full of needles with steroids and an anesthetic, the neurologist will check out your brain's neuronal activity, the chiropractor will adjust you, and the orthopedist or neurosurgeon will look for places to start his or her incision. Even so-called comprehensive spine-care centers are invariably unidirectional in the care they give. Put simply, depending on who is treating you, you're likely to get one type of treatment that may or may not help you. And what if your pain isn't even originating from your back?

It happens more than you can imagine: Back pain may actually not be coming from the back. A study of 368 back pain patients published in the journal *Spine* in 2009 found that a full 35 percent experienced back pain from unknown or so-called nonspinal pain generators. Even MRIs can be misleading, because abnormalities, such as degenerating discs, can be seen on scans for virtually everyone over the age of thirty regardless of whether they have pain. In fact, so many things seemingly unrelated to the back may cause back pain. Examples include benign and malignant tumors, ovarian cysts, uterine fibroids, endometriosis, kidney infections, kidney/gallstones, aortic aneurysms, depression, Lyme disease, vitamin D deficiency, and shingles. Side effects from certain medications such as those used to lower cholesterol may also mimic back pain. This is why I will stress the need for an accurate diagnosis. It's important to know where your back pain is coming from. And to know that typically calls for a spinal *generalist*—not a specialist.

A spinal generalist is someone who is willing to take a comprehensive history and full exam, and review or prescribe the necessary diagnostic tests in order to make a definitive diagnosis before suggesting the treatment plan most likely to suit your particular diagnosis. Such generalists are, unfortunately, lacking in the medical system.

All too often, I see patients who are still suffering after failed courses of physical therapy, chiropractic care, epidural steroid injections, facet blocks, and surgery. They come to me after they've been to a handful of other doctors or therapists. When I ask these patients about their diagnoses, they consistently say "low back pain," which is akin to someone saying he has had extensive treatment for a "rash." A rash, like low back pain, is not enough of a precise diagnosis to prescribe effective treatment. Is the rash a minor case of poison ivy or a potentially serious condition such as psoriasis? Is your back pain from a benign muscle spasm or is it an early sign of a spinal tumor? Here again I need to stress two points. The first is that it's imperative to obtain as accurate a diagnosis as possible for effective treatment. And second, an accurate diagnosis is not always possible even in the best of hands.

What all this means is that you, the patient, need to educate yourself about your particular problem. I suspect that it has always been true to some extent, but the need to advocate for your medical care never seemed more urgent than it does today. My own daily battles, as I try to be the best doctor that I can be, are a constant reminder of the importance of self-advocacy. I deal with insurance companies that want to limit the services I feel my patients need and deserve, I negotiate with diagnostic imaging centers that cut corners in the quality of the tests they perform, and I wrestle with hospitals that prefer to discharge my patients before I feel they are ready. This shortens the "average length of stay," which translates to a more robust reimbursement. I also have to contend with some colleagues who will shortchange patients because of lack of time or interest, and others who are familiar with only one form of treatment, and therefore treat all lower back pain the same way—often ineffectively.

Anatomy of Pain

Unlike most back pain books, the emphasis here is not on the anatomy of the spine, but on the anatomy of *pain*. In the next chapter we're going to take a tour of those parts of the spine that most often cause pain—the pain generators. These represent key anatomical elements in making an accurate diagnosis and the first step on the road to treatment. We'll also begin to explore the biology of pain, which has both physiological and psychological components.

THERE ARE ONLY a limited number of specific anatomical sites that cause pain in almost 100 percent of patients. We will call these the Six Pain Generators. Once you have a better understanding of your pain generators, you'll see that they correspond to a small number of common diagnoses.

Pain is most often a *perception*, and not a sensation, at least not in the same way as seeing, smelling, and hearing are. Both mind and body must be explored to form a complete understanding of the anatomy of pain. Pain is physical and emotional, acute and chronic. Right now a lot of research and experimentation is being conducted to sort out the uncertainties in pain medicine, and it appears to be only a matter of time before pain can be managed more effectively.

Because pain hinges on perception, it fails to have certain defined, universal parameters that apply to everyone. With no measurable thresholds from a scientific standpoint, pain often must be described according to a scale of 1 to 10. My "level 6" pain, however, will be different from yours. And since pain is hard to calculate, it makes the diagnosis of back pain in particular more of an art than a science.

Why Surgery Is Far from a Sure Thing

When people ask me about the benefits to surgery, I am cautious in my reply. Given the richly gray area I just described that is back pain, you can begin to see how surgery can be a tenuous proposition unless you know exactly what's wrong and there's a known—operable—solution.

Lest I be accused of giving spinal surgeons like myself a pass, let me point out that the indications for spinal surgery have broadened to the point that the number of such surgeries has grown exponentially, a fact I pointed out in the introduction. I wish I could say that the success rate has grown at the same rate.

The strange fact is that the most invasive treatments for spinal surgery, from injections to complex spinal surgeries, are not regulated by the FDA in the same way that medication is. (Case in point: In a commentary published in 2013 in the *Journal of the American Medical Association*, researchers from the Netherlands point out that there is almost no evidence that injection therapy eases most people's pain long term, even after multiple injections. Other studies show that injections don't dramatically reduce the likelihood of back surgery later.) Such procedures, be they injections or surgery, do not undergo the same rigorous standards for a number of reasons, one of which is that it's very difficult to find a group of patients who are similar enough for researchers to suitably compare outcomes of the same problem in patients with and without surgery. Unlike a drug test, in which one group receives the drug and the other gets the placebo, or dummy pill, studies in surgery that adhere to the gold standard (i.e., randomized, double-blind controlled studies) are just not possible. Nor is it ethical to have a placebo group in whom an incision would be made, but the operation itself would not be performed. And in this regard, surgery may always remain more art than science.

For some patients, the need for spine surgery may be legitimate, but even when the procedure is a success, it rarely dispels 100 percent of back pain. As with so many things in life, lasting success often comes about through a combination of approaches. Each strategy may reduce pain by just 10 or 20 percent (from the perspective of the patient), but those percentages can add up, so that ultimately your pain is cut back by as much as 70 or 80 percent.

When Jenna first came to me, she had good reason to be skeptical. A longtime back pain sufferer, she'd undergone spinal fusion (a technique we'll explore in chapter 5) at the hands of another doctor to treat spinal stenosis, a narrowing of the channel through which spinal nerves pass. The surgery was intended to fix the problem and silence the pain. But after about a month, she was practically suicidal again with intolerable jolts of pain down her left leg and unrelenting back-aches. Her surgery had failed to remedy her back.

Jenna is not alone in her relapse experience. Nearly 600,000 Americans opt for back operations each year, but for many like Jenna, surgery is just an empty promise. A recent study published in the journal *Spine* in 2011 shows that in many cases surgery can backfire, leaving patients in even more pain. The statistics are quite sober-ing. Researchers from the University of Cincinnati College of Medi-cine, Meharry Medical College in Nashville, and the University of Kentucky College of Medicine reviewed records of 1,450 patients in the Ohio Bureau of Workers' Compensation database who had diag-noses of disc degeneration, disc herniation, or radiculopathy, a nerve condition that features tingling and weakness of the limbs. Half of the patients had surgery to fuse two or more vertebrae in hopes of curing low back pain. The other half had no surgery, even though they had comparable diagnoses.

After two years, just 26 percent of those who had surgery returned to work. That's compared to 67 percent of patients who didn't have surgery. In what might be the most troubling study finding, research-ers determined that there was a 41 percent increase in the use of pow-erful painkillers, specifically opiates, in those who had surgery. The study provides clear evidence that for many patients with back in-juries, fusion surgeries designed to alleviate pain from degenerating discs don't work. It's important to note that these were work-related in-juries, which can entail a multitude of compounding factors aside from the actual pain. The potential benefits reaped from filing a workers' compensation claim, for example, muddy the waters when doctors try to figure out the root cause of someone's pain and treatment.

Not all was lost for Jenna, whose pain wasn't instigated by an ac-tual work-related injury. But like so many fellow sufferers, she had to accept that her back pain wouldn't be cured by a magic bullet. She would need to scale back her expectations, but with the right treatments, she could ease her pain and enjoy life again. Once I explained to Jenna the reality of her situation, we worked as a team to put together a non-invasive course of therapy. She learned to respect her back and to find ways to avoid irritating the nerves in her spine. She began an exercise program designed specifically to strengthen the muscles in her lower back and abdomen so that her spine would get better support. She also cleaned up her diet, which allowed her to lose the excess weight that aggravated her symptoms. We'll be visiting all of these options in upcoming steps when we explore the choices you have to match your diagnosis. You'll learn what to try, and how to design your own personal protocol.

To some degree, a few aches and pains are a part of life, and a consequence of getting older in a world where medicine can help us to outperform how long our bodies were naturally built to last. We can get new knees when our long-distance-running habits catch up to us. We can have cataracts removed and clear away the cobwebs that set up camp in our old eyes. We can take hormones, if we so choose, to outrun the marches of middle age when we reach meno- and andro-pause. But we can't get a new spine when something goes wrong back there. While it's true that we can be very successful in treating an assortment of age-related maladies, we can't do quite the same for our backs.

Yet if there's any good news to embrace, it's this: Resolving your back pain starts with you. Back pain may be one of the more elusive and exceedingly exasperating challenges to overcome (and to manage when it's chronic), but it doesn't have to be a life sentence. Thankfully, we live in a time when there's an enormous amount of information to mine and make relevant to you and your back. So, whether you find a total cure or a pain management tool will depend largely on how you utilize and employ that information. And with all of that in mind, let's begin the process of breaking your back's secret code by taking a tour of its geography that can elicit pain.

ACTION PLAN

- Make sure that you answer the questionnaire starting on page 4 as honestly as you can and to the best of your ability. If you're unsure how to answer questions about family medical history, for example, don't be afraid to ask! Did your mom have disc disease in her fifties? Is there bone cancer on your dad's side of the family? Has your sister already been treated for osteoporosis and osteoarthritis? Creating a family history of health conditions that could lead to back pain is important.
- Record how long your back pain has lasted. Are you reading this with pain for less than six weeks or do you think you're dealing with chronic pain that's gone on far too long—more than six weeks?
- Be open-minded about the approach to your care. You may think you can pin your back pain on a single culprit for which a single remedy exists, but we have to consider more than just anatomical issues and concrete cures.

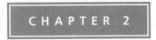

CHAPTER 2

Decoding the Geography of Pain

T HE ODD SENSATION STARTED in her lower back, a little to the right. An avid runner, Kathryn chalked it up to her long jaunt that morning down to the beach and back. She popped some ibuprofen to try to settle the dull sensation. Later that day, the ache had progressed to the point that Kathryn found herself resting her hand over her lower back for a quick self-massage as she maneuvered around the kitchen to prepare for a dinner party. She wasn't the type to be easily convinced of something going awfully wrong with her physically, and she'd had her fair share of sports-related injuries. In fact, the feeling resembled one of a pinched or agitated nerve, and she assumed this could be another sciatic episode. Or perhaps she had strained a muscle. Whatever it was, she didn't think twice about her growing discomfort and lower back's tenderness. If she worried about anything, it was that this escalating soreness would disrupt her run the next morning, and she'd have to take a few days off.

By the time her dinner guests left and Kathryn was preparing for bed, she sensed that something wasn't right. She took another round of ibuprofen and decided that a good long sleep—off her feet—would be the cure.

At one o'clock in the morning, Kathryn awakened with a high fever, chills, and a serious sweat. She forgot about the backache and now thought that maybe she was suffering from food poisoning, vowing to grin and bear it. She did her best to sleep through the night, but it wasn't easy. The sweating was profuse at times and in addition to wild swings in her body's temperature from low to high, she experienced episodes of violent whole-body shaking that got even her husband concerned. By morning, it was clear that whatever Kathryn was fighting wasn't going to go away soon enough. It was time to call the doctor.

Flash forward a couple of hours. Kathryn is sitting in her primary-care physician's office, sore and beaten up from the dramatic symptoms that had taken over her life in the previous twelve hours. Everything hurt, including her joints and muscles. Her overall discomfort eclipsed the throbbing ache still in her lower back. As her doctor scrolled through her medical history and asked a series of questions to help nail down exactly what could be wrong with her, he went as far as to ask if she'd traveled to South America lately and perhaps picked up dengue fever. And then Kathryn remembered how it all started: with a nagging twinge in her lower back, just to the right.

"You should be in the emergency room," he told her. "This has nothing to do with your back." His instincts were right on target. That afternoon, after giving Kathryn a powerful dose of antibiotics, it was confirmed that she had a case of acute bacterial pyelonephritis— a bacterial infection in her kidneys that was making its way to her bloodstream. It took her two weeks to recover and get back on the running trails.

A case like Kathryn's is dramatic but short and to the point: The diagnosis can be made relatively quickly and a remedy is waiting. I learned about her story through her physician, who happens to be a colleague. Kathryn's case occurred the same week I saw a patient with similarly agonizing flank pain radiating from her lower back. My patient's story had a different ending, though. It turned out that she had a kidney stone, which was confirmed by a CT scan and treated with a course of pain medication until the stone passed. Though she first said that her main problem was "back pain," I later learned that her pain was localized more toward her flank than the small of her back. This instantly ruled out a lot of potential culprits of back pain and clued me in to a host of conditions that mimic low back pain, including kidney stones. Problems with the kidneys can cause back pain, since the kidneys are located in that general region of the body. The kidneys themselves are perched high on the back, just under the lower ribs, but complications such as stones moving down and out of them or an infection in the ureter can feel like back pain. For this reason, it's important to map pain's geography and identify the difference between, for example, pain isolated to the lower back and pain that's felt on one's side. In turn, this helps a doctor figure out what's actually causing the pain.

For both of these women, though, the turning point in their cases came when we doctors could isolate exactly where their pain originated—to get to the source as quickly as possible and then hunt down further clues to arrive at an accurate diagnosis. Kathryn didn't have the luxury of time, given her rapidly blooming bacterial infection, which could have done serious damage not only to her kidneys but elsewhere as it moved through her bloodstream. Had she not recalled that seemingly minor pain "in her back," and been specific about its odd sensation over "to the side," accompanied by a fever and chills, it may have taken much longer to pinpoint the offending cause as she awaited a litany of clinical and laboratory tests.

The goal of this chapter is to help you identify the source of your pain. Where is your pain emanating from, exactly? How does your pain match up with one or more of the six most common anatomical origins for pain, which are called the back's pain generators? The answers to these questions will help you decode the real reason for your pain, and then take the proper steps to treat it successfully.

This is the first step in our journey. It's simple: If you can't peg your pain to a specific pain generator, then you can't begin to effectively cure or manage it. To start, let's talk first about the basics of back biomechanics.

Back Biomechanics

Understanding the mechanical importance of the spine is really no different from knowing how the liver plays a role in digestion or the

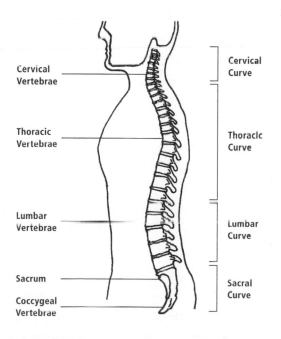

The spinal (vertebral) column is divided into four main sections, with the lumbar curve being the anatomical "lower back." The image above shows the various parts of the spinal column, each of which can play a part in a pain generator.

lungs manage respiration. By the time our heart started beating for the very first time at about three weeks in utero, our spine's development was well under way. When you were just an embryo your cells were rapidly developing their striking segmented pattern of a human spine, which now allows you to stand erect and walk.

As a whole, the spinal column serves three chief functions: (1) to protect the spinal cord from damage and thereby secure the brain's neurological connections with the rest of the body; (2) to facilitate weight bearing, which is why the vertebrae—the individual bones in the spinal column—increase in size toward the bottom; and (3) to provide motion, which is largely the responsibility of the intervertebral discs, which are between each of the vertebrae. Each disc also forms a cartilaginous joint to allow slight movement of the vertebrae, and acts as a hinge to hold the vertebrae together. As you can see from the diagram on the previous page, the spinal column is divided into four main sections. Mobility is greatest at the cervical curve in your neck, which permits you to quickly move your head up, down, to the right, and to the left; it's least mobile at the thoracic curve, where the ribs decrease mobility and increase stability, thereby protecting your lungs and heart. The combination of these three features is what allows us to perform truly extraordinary physical feats, from pole vaulting and mountain climbing to the simple pleasures of bending, twisting, and engaging in everyday activities, while protecting the spinal cord at the same time.

The spinal cord can be thought of as the electrical highway that allows for two-way communication between the brain and the peripheral nerves. In its simplest description, the brain controls the body's movements, both voluntary and involuntary, and the peripheral nerves inform the brain about the status of the body's environment.

Your brain is a chief command center: All your nerves, joints, and bones, and even your skin, send messages via the spinal cord to your brain. Which is why neurosurgeons like me always look for motor and sensory functions in an exam, as they can help clue us in to what's going on in the back. Can the person walk a straight line, maintain good balance, and catch a ball? All of these activities require high-functioning sensory and motor skills, which are the skills that allow us to organize and integrate different sensations quickly from the environment (the sensory part) to then move effectively within that environment (the motor part).

Thanks to your spinal cord's highway of message transmission, if you were to close your eyes you'd still be able to know whether or not you're standing up or sitting down, whether the room is hot or cold, and if there's a breeze blowing on your face. If someone pushes against you, specialized receptors spring into action and tell you how big or small of a "pushback" you need to execute to respond accordingly. One important feature of the spinal cord to keep in mind is that it's a two-way highway. There's an *afferent* and an *efferent* side to it. Afferent, or sensory, neurons carry nerve impulses from receptors or sense organs toward the central nervous system so that the body can produce a response; efferent, or motor, neurons go the opposite direction—they carry nerve impulses away from the central nervous system to effectors such as the muscles.

Don't panic. I won't ask you to distinguish among different types of nerves or figure out the anatomy of the nervous system. But I do want you to appreciate the intricacies of your body's mechanics and come to learn how pain generators have different and identifiable characteristics. The Six Pain Generators, after all, have everything to do with what's going on in the spinal cord. Once you have a basic understanding of the cord's prime purpose and functionality, you'll be able to quickly grasp the meaning and significance of the main pain generators.

The checklist you filled out starting on page 4 summarizes the key features of different types of pain generators and can give your doctor a head start in diagnosing your pain. As you read through the description of each pain generator in this section, highlight any piece of information that resonates with you and your particular pain.

Location! Location! Location!

It's a straightforward question: *Where does it hurt?*

Whether it's shooting leg pain or simply an aching muscle, we can usually attribute a specific symptom to one or more pain generators. This is why it's critical that you identify your symptoms. Do you have back pain or leg pain? Is your pain on the left or right side? Is the pain accompanied by weight loss or a fever? Does the pain occur when you stand, stretch, or sit? Is it worse in the morning and better at night—or vice versa? Does it intensify if you cough, sneeze, or move your bowels? These are just a smattering of the clues that can help you identify the source. Start thinking about them so that I can help you pinpoint the symptoms and then identify the potential or actual pain generator.

Anatomy is basically human geography. Since very few of the hundreds of structures that make up the low back cause pain, I had to decide how much geography you really needed to know. Imagine asking someone for directions from Boston to New York City and receiving a map of the entire United States. It's interesting, but too much information to actually be helpful. Pain patients need to know only which parts of their lower-back anatomy most often cause pain.

So, we begin this journey by looking for a correlation between the symptom and a specific anatomical location. These locations are not

---

THE THREE QUESTIONS

1. Where exactly is the pain? If you haven't done so already, use the model on page 6 to draw your pain.
2. How would you describe the pain (e.g., throbbing, dull, sharp, burning, shooting, constant, intermittent)?
3. What makes the pain better and what makes it worse?

random. There are approximately Six primary Pain Generators in the low back that are responsible for the majority of back pain. Let's get to know them.

Pain Generator #1: Muscles

You may recognize yourself if you are the person who is walking around with your arms behind you as you hold your back, seeking relief. The area may actually feel warm to the touch; you may even have a tendency to rub or massage the area, which makes it feel better. You may also notice that bending forward also makes it feel better, and so does your position, especially when you lie down. Sometimes you may remember exactly how the symptoms began: The pain started after you played eighteen holes of golf. But most often the pain develops insidiously, and only in retrospect would you remember that day on the golf course.

Injury to the muscles of the back is the single most common cause of low back pain. Your back muscles—also called the paraspinal muscles—are an amazing group. As with the other 320 pairs of skeletal muscles in your body, they support your spine and provide the force of movement between all the vertebrae and the rest of the skeleton. In all likelihood, this type of back pain is caused by tears and strains in the muscle tissues attached to the bones of your back. Although millions of us suffer from low back pain, there is, in my experience, no typical muscular–low-back-pain patient. I see it in lean, muscular athletes as well as in couch potatoes. In fact, I put the majority of people who rake leaves into the same category as the stereotypical "weekend warrior." Chances are they don't exercise regularly; they haven't stretched and their muscles are cold and stiff. Most people warm up before exercising, but how many give any thought to stretching or taking a warm shower before setting out for a day of raking leaves? Skeletal muscles are very responsive to use and disuse.

IS YOUR PAIN COMING FROM A MUSCLE?

SIGNS OF A MUSCULAR PAIN GENERATOR: Your pain is confined to your back. Your pain goes away without much treatment after a few days or weeks (it can be very painful at the start, but subsides over time). You experience some relief with ice packs and over-the-counter anti-inflammatories.

COMMON CAUSES: physical trauma/injury.

QUESTIONS TO ASK YOURSELF: Is the area warm to the touch? Can you feel an actual knot or area of spasm in the muscle? Does the pain increase when you stretch the muscle? Have you been engaging in a new sport or activity recently? Do you have any soreness specific to a single muscle area, such as your hamstrings or quadriceps?

If you answer yes to any of these questions, your pain could be originating from a muscle or soft tissue (see pain generator #2) in your back. This is typically a diagnosis of exclusion (other pain generators have been ruled out) and your doctor will likely start you on a course of treatment in seeking relief, which can include muscle relaxants, non-steroidal anti-inflammatories, physical therapy, massage, deep heat, and electrical stimulation. Relief within a relatively short time period from these therapies further confirms the diagnosis.

The recurrence rate of muscular low back pain is high. In my experience, this is because the folks who misuse their bodies tend to repeat the tasks or behaviors that aggravate their backs. At times this relates to the type of physical work that some people do, whether it's being a laborer, or a pianist who sits hunched over the keyboard. These back pain sufferers can benefit from improved body mechanics and strength building using some of the techniques I'll recommend later in this book.

Those that are vigorously exercised tend to enlarge and grow stronger. Conversely, a muscle that is not used undergoes atrophy, decreasing in size and strength and increasing the risk for injury.

In addition to strains and tears to these muscles, spasms may also develop, indirectly causing injury. A muscle spasm, or cramp, is simply a tightening of a muscle that fails to relax. Spasms usually occur as a protective reflex upon injury to the spine in order to reduce motion in the area that could result in further damage. If you've ever experienced a prolonged muscle spasm, you may also notice an uncomfortable burning sensation. This is the result of lactic acid building up in your muscles, a waste product produced by the chemical reaction inside muscle cells. The main reason why lactic acid accumulates is that when the muscles contract, the small blood vessels traveling through the muscles are pinched off, creating a bottleneck where lactic acid can collect (just like a tube pinched between your thumb and finger). When the muscle relaxes, the lactic acid is eventually washed away by fresh blood flowing into the muscle as those blood vessels open up again. Athletes who occasionally overtax their muscles in physical training or competition are very familiar with the achy sensation of excess lactic acid sitting in their muscles, which adequate rest typically cures.

Pain Generator #2: Soft Tissue

Soft tissue inflammation is a major cause of low back pain. Soft tissue injuries are very difficult to distinguish from muscular injuries and even harder to diagnose and treat. That's because what we usually refer to as soft tissue pain is related to injuries to the tendons and ligaments. While there's a tendency in medicine to lump ligaments and tendons together—both are connective tissue made from collagen cells produced by proteins—they are very different. Ligaments are strong, fibrous soft tissues that firmly attach bones to bones. Ligaments secure each of the vertebrae and surround each of the discs. A tendon, on the other hand, links muscle to bone and is really an anchoring point for a muscle. It's actually more accurate to group tendons and muscles together since the tendon is the "stroma," or supporting framework, of the entire muscle-tendon unit. The Achilles tendon, for example, attaches our calf muscle to our anklebone. On the other hand, the anterior cruciate ligament (ACL) holds the calf and thighbone together at the knee joint.

Another important difference between tendons and ligaments is that tendons are active and ligaments are passive. Many muscle groups that are responsible for flexing, extending, and rotating the waist, as well as moving the lower extremities, connect to the lumbar spine through tendon insertions. Tendons are part of our complex neuro-muscular system and they detect the degree of stretch and electri-cally transmit that message to muscles, which in concert allows them to flex smoothly. Ligaments, on the other hand, carry no electrical charges. Ligaments are tough and sturdy, and since they can't sig-nificantly expand, they are not involved in stretching. They simply cushion and protect joints affected by muscle movement. Because of the ligaments' supportive role, elasticity is actually not a desirable quality. One notable exception to this is the ligamentum flavum, a stretchy ligament that is found from the top to the bottom of the spinal column. Because its job is to protect the spinal cord and nerves in the enveloping spinal column, it doesn't hold anything in place or stop any joints from dislocating. It gives with all the movements of the spinal column.

Damaged ligaments have a direct impact on mobility because they can cause a misalignment of the bones that the ligament(s) formerly held in place. The muscles connected to the joint can still react to electrical stimulus, but the joint itself cannot provide support for the movement. Both ligaments and tendons must be in working order to provide pain-free mobility and other functions. Every connective tissue in your back, including your ligaments and tendons, if stretched

IS YOUR PAIN COMING FROM SOFT TISSUE?

SIGNS OF A SOFT TISSUE PAIN GENERATOR: sensation of heat or warmth in the pain area, swelling, pain that accompanies performing a specific activity or movement, some relief upon taking an over-the-counter anti-inflammatory (e.g., Advil or Aleve). Note: Soft tissue damage can be difficult to distinguish from muscle pain. Only your doctor can help you differentiate between a *strain* and a *sprain*. Muscle strains happen when the muscle fibers are abnormally stretched or torn. A sprain, on the other hand, occurs when the ligaments—the tough bands of tissue that hold bones together—are abnormally stretched and then torn from their attachments. Both injuries exhibit similar symptoms, and their treatment and prognosis are the same. With one exception: If you tear a ligament from its attachment, recovery can take much longer than if you had just sprained it or strained a muscle. Severe soft tissue damage requires a lengthy healing process and in some rare cases, surgery.

COMMON CAUSES: trauma/injury, improper body mechanics (e.g., improper lifting or bending).

QUESTIONS TO ASK YOURSELF: Have you recently participated in an activity that can cause injury or that you haven't done in a long time? Did you "sprain" your back while bending or lifting a heavy object?

If you answered yes to any of these questions, your pain could be originating from soft tissue, and a doctor can help you ensure it's not from a muscle.

or torn, has the potential to cause pain. And it's challenging to identify which of the tendons or ligaments is the actual pain generator because they are poorly visualized in imaging studies. What does help me distinguish between muscular low back pain and what's known as ligamentous or tendinous (soft tissue) pain is that the latter tends to be localized to a specific, usually identifiable area in your lower spine, not generalized discomfort that is typical of muscular low back pain.

Pain Generator #3: Bones

Pain of bony origin must be diagnosed quickly, though it's relatively much easier to spot than pain of muscular or soft tissue origin. When the pain is associated with trauma, such as an automobile accident, the cause may be obvious. It may represent a mild break (benign fracture),

---

IS YOUR PAIN COMING FROM A BONE?

SIGNS OF A BONE PAIN GENERATOR: extreme pain in one particular area rather than generalized pain, "point tenderness" (when you press on the area in question, you experience extreme pain), difficulty with movement.

COMMON CAUSES: trauma/injury, cancer, osteopenia/osteoporosis.

QUESTIONS TO ASK YOURSELF: Have you been injured or been in a recent accident? Do you have a history of cancer or osteopenia/osteoporosis? Have you ever had a bone density scan that shows the signs of reduced bone mass, called osteopenia, or the more severe form called osteoporosis? Are you over the age of fifty-five?

If you answered yes to any combination of these questions, then your pain could be originating from the vertebrae itself. This is when imaging with X-rays, MRIs, and bone scans is key to identifying why the bones of the vertebrae are causing pain. Any number of culprits may be to blame, including a tumor, compression fracture, or bone cyst. If cancer is suspected, further tests must be performed to determine which kind (e.g., bone cancer or metastatic cancer that originated elsewhere in the body) is resulting in the backbone pain.

but it may also represent a more serious break that has the potential to compromise the spinal cord or the nerve roots. In the elderly, especially women with osteoporosis, it may further represent a compression fracture. With an aging population, hardly a week goes by without a call from the emergency room to treat a compression fracture. Of even greater concern is the fact that bone pain is one of the signs of cancer. If I'm called in to treat severe pain on the oncology floor, I immediately start to think of metastatic bone cancer, particularly if the patient has already been diagnosed with breast or prostate cancer, since these frequently spread to the bone. Treatment in such a situation will depend on the nature of the tumor and may entail chemotherapy, radiation therapy, and/or surgery. The treatments in general are well established with varying degrees of success.

A Note About the Physiology of Pain

As you've just learned, the primary pain generators of the lumbar/ mechanical low back are muscle, soft tissue, and bone. These tissues, like all body tissues, have connections to nerve fibers, which terminate in sites that act as special receptors to respond to changes in their environment. If these changes are interpreted as harmful, then they send messages along the nerve fibers to the spinal cord and ultimately to the brain. The brain interprets these messages as painful, and you then respond. The simplest example of this is the reflex arc.

You may remember from elementary biology the image of a young man putting his hand too close to the cooking stove and the receptors in the periphery. In this case his hand senses this dangerous change in the environment and within nanoseconds a message is sent through the spinal cord to his brain, where almost instantaneously another message is sent back down. Without conscious thought, the boy removes his hand. This is the reflex arc in action.

For most of us mechanical low back pain sufferers, this is not the type of pain we usually experience. Our pain is typically not the sharp pain or acute pain experienced when we touch the frying pan handle or step on a tack. (And a reflexive action won't remove the pain, either.) Much to the contrary, and to our dismay, mechanical low back pain is usually more insidious—a deep, annoying, irritating discomfort that can make the activities of daily living a miserable experience. The reason for this is that there are a wide variety of receptors that respond to different noxious stimuli.

The pain generators we have discussed so far are those that respond to tissue injury, be it muscular, soft, or bone. When those receptors stay "on," sending pain signals to the brain, we experience them as chronic pain. Unlike the hand touching the hot frying pain, the tissue keeps signaling pain to the brain. This is also why treatments such as ice, aspirin, or non-steroidal anti-inflammatories can be so effective. These decrease the inflammatory response—the chemicals the body produces in response to the injury—which in turn modifies and decreases the pain message to the brain. These are important clues, because if your pain responds to these types of treatments, it's probably because your pain is related to soft tissue injury.

Before we move on, I want to point out that one attribute that the first three pain generators have in common is they tend to produce pain localized to the lower back, what we call axial or mechanical pain. The next three pain generators often produce pain that radiates down one or both legs, what is known as radicular pain. This difference is especially important as we hunt for clues to your particular diagnosis.

Pain Generator #4: Discs

The intervertebral discs are soft, rubbery pads that serve as "cushions" between each vertebral body. They help to minimize the impact of stress forces on the spinal column. Each disc is said to resemble a jelly doughnut with a central, softer component called the nucleus pulposus and a surrounding outer ring (annulus fibrosus). But in all honesty, when asked about the consistency of the disc material, instead of jelly I compare it to the artificial crabmeat sold at a deli. It's fibrous and resilient. Next time you're at the supermarket, stop by the deli counter and examine the product. It will give you a good sense of what your disc looks and feels like.

Two other observations you can make while at the deli counter: (1) The crabmeat has striations, or fissures. Remember this image when we discuss the concept of annular tears or tears within the disc material itself, which are frequently a diagnostic hallmark of changes within the disc that are produced by either age or trauma and cause pain. And (2) note that there is no blood supply in the fiber cartilage. That's because the blood vessels receded from the discs during embryogenesis. This lack of a blood supply is probably one factor that contributes to the development of degenerative disc material in almost all of us and helps explain the discs' inability to regenerate adequately when injured.

In fact, a significant number of you may have chronic low back pain from degenerative disc disease. The characteristic pain is located in the midline. It is frequently worse with weight bearing, improves with lying down, and worsens again with vigorous activity, especially physically demanding tasks. To some degree, degenerative disc pain inevitably afflicts most of us, especially if we are sixty or older, and for some the pain will develop sooner.

Simple X rays frequently give indications of this diagnosis. The most common finding is an obvious reduction in disc height. An MRI almost always confirms these reductions in disc height and documents the fissures, or annular tears, in the disc material itself. Sometimes there is so little disc material remaining that two vertebrae are touching or almost touching. In that case, the MRI may also demonstrate inflammatory changes within the bone itself. In another chapter, we'll discuss further diagnostic tests needed to confirm the diagnosis and the treatment options if you carry this diagnosis.

Most patients with discogenic disease don't have pain radiating down their leg because no matter how degenerated the disc material

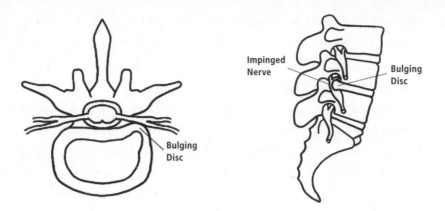

A herniated disc (cross section and side view). A disc herniates, or ruptures, when part of the center nucleus pushes through the outer edge of the disc and back toward the spinal canal. This puts pressure on the nerves. Spinal nerves are very sensitive to even slight amounts of pressure, which can result in pain, numbness, or weakness in one or both legs.

has become, it has remained within the confines of disc space. The material has not bulged, herniated, or become extruded to the point where it presses against the nerve that then causes pain to travel down one or both legs. But of course this can and does happen.

Discs are numbered in reference to the vertebrae between which they lie. Therefore, the L3-L4 disc (i.e., lumbar 3-lumbar 4) is the one between the L3 and L4 vertebra, and the L5-S1 (i.e., lumbar 5-sacrum 1) disc is the disc between the fifth lumbar vertebra and the sacrum. Considering the fancy Latin names that early anatomists used, I think this designation for the location of the discs is quite straightforward and functional.

There are actually differences among bulging, herniated, and extruded discs, though these terms are sometimes used interchangeably and many people resort to using the catch-all phrase "slipped disc" to refer to any one of these conditions. Discs are essentially elliptically shaped and made of two components. The outer is called the annulus fibrosus. As it implies, these are more fibrotic, or thicker, fibers that encase the central fibers, which are less fibrotic. A disc *bulge* usually implies that the outer, fibrotic fibers have bulged out. Usually, the pressure on the disc reaches such magnitude that it weakens a portion of the disc wall. Some of you may be old enough to remember when your car tires would do this. If this weakened wall actually develops an opening so that the inner core can herniate through, it's called a *herniation*. It follows, then, that if the portion that herniates through the annulus is no longer in continuity with the fibers from which it came, it's labeled an *extrusion*.

Keep in mind that the size of the extrusion is not always directly related to the amount of pain you are experiencing. A small extrusion can cause severe radicular pain, whereas a large extrusion can cause minimal or no symptoms. It depends a lot on whether the extruded or herniated disc fragment is compressing a nerve root, and sometimes it also depends on the size of your spinal canal. A small fragment is more likely to cause symptoms if you were born with a small spinal canal.

Conventional wisdom would suggest that the majority of people who experience herniated discs earn their living through some form of intense physical activity or heavy labor. It is thought that they have done something that has gone beyond the disc's ability to absorb the force. But a herniated disc can happen to anyone. I see many patients who live sedentary lives or exercise sporadically and yet they also develop disc disease. I recently operated on a lawyer and weekend runner whose herniated disc likely resulted from many years of wear and tear, and not a specific traumatic event or recent run. This is an example of how the constant pounding of running wore out his annulus, which again is the outer wall of the intervertebral disc, causing the nucleus pulposus to extrude and press against the sciatic nerve. On the other hand, I have another patient with a herniated disc whose injury occurred after she tried unsuccessfully to install a very large air conditioner in her bedroom window. And then there are those patients who suffer herniated discs without any obvious cause. Some evidence suggests, however, that herniated discs run in families, which means there is likely an unidentified genetic component.

Back Water

IN CHILDREN AND young adults, discs have high water content. As you age, the water content in the discs naturally decreases and the discs become less flexible. They then begin to shrink and the spaces between the vertebrae get narrower, making you vulnerable to a "slipped" or herniated disc.

IS YOUR PAIN COMING FROM A DISC?

SIGNS OF A DISC PAIN GENERATOR: The pain comes on suddenly and is usually one-sided (unilateral leg pain), increasing with coughing or sneezing, or allowing you to literally draw a diagram of the course of your pain radiating like a bolt of lightning—that is, you can trace where the pain starts to where it lands in your thigh or at the front of your toes. Other signs include the following: you are more comfortable with your knees bent (particularly lying down); you notice numbness or tingling in your leg, foot, or toes; you may notice even the loss of some strength in your leg, foot, or toes; and the possibility that you notice a subtle or obvious loss of control over bowel and bladder function.

COMMON CAUSES: trauma/injury, improper lifting, sudden pressure (which can be slight), repetitive strenuous activities, weakened discs from age or other medical conditions.

QUESTIONS TO ASK YOURSELF: Do you have a family history of degenerative disc disease? Have you had an injury lately? Does pain increase when you cough or sneeze? Do you have weakness in one leg that causes you to drag your foot? Do you experience tingling (a pins-and-needles sensation) or numbness in one arm? Can you draw the pain going down the leg on the model on page 6? Do you smoke? Are you overweight? (Smoking and carrying extra weight, which put an added strain on your discs, are common risk factors.) Have you noticed difficulty in controlling your bowels and bladder?

If you answered yes to any combination of these questions, then your pain could be originating from a disc. Imaging tests can help with the diagnosis, and treatment will depend on the extent of the damage and how it has manifested itself. Chiropractic care, steroids, NSAIDs, physical therapy, and sometimes surgery have all been used to treat herniated discs. (For more specifics about treatment options, see chapter 5.) If you do experience numbness, loss of strength, or a tingling sensation in your leg, foot, or toes, I recommend that you get immediate medical attention.

Some Things That I'm Thinking About

Each one of the nerve roots that exits your lumbar spine goes to the specific muscle or muscles, a general area of skin, and a specific reflex. This means that when I examine a patient and discover that he has weakness in his right quadriceps and a loss of the reflex in his right knee, but then I look at the MRI and it shows a good-size herniated disc at L5-S1, it's unlikely that the disc at that level is causing the patient's symptoms. Why? Because the quads and patellar reflexes are usually controlled by the L3-L4 disc—not the L5-S1. Remember: The exam and the imaging studies must jibe with each other. The same would be true if I saw a herniated disc at L3-L4 on the left side, because again it's unlikely that a left-sided herniation will cause right-sided symptoms! Although I don't expect you to know or study which spinal discs correlate with which muscles or other anatomy (that's the job of your doctor), I stress this because you are becoming an educated patient and you need to appreciate these pitfalls that can happen in the diagnosing. Put simply, make sure that your symptoms and your injury match! It's the only way to get a correct diagnosis.

Pain Generator #5: Facets

"I just bent over to pick something up and my back went and I couldn't move!"

The usual attack of acute back pain involving facet joints occurs suddenly and with no warning. The facets are the lubricating joints located between each vertebra and that allow for the movement between individual bones. Without the facet joints, you would not have flexibility in your spine, and you could move only in very straight, stiff motions. The facet joints are known as synovial joints, and are similar in structure and function to a knee or elbow, since they allow for movement between two bones. In a synovial joint, the ends of the bones are covered with articular cartilage, a shiny, very smooth, almost frictionless material that allows the bones to glide against one another.

Facet joint injuries can appear dramatic, leaving patients in so much discomfort that they cannot move very well. I once saw a woman with terrible, numbing pain running down her right leg. Even without an MRI, I suspected, going by the nature of her symptoms

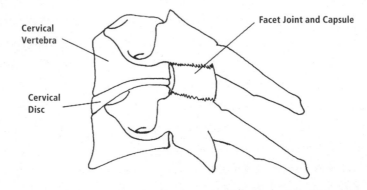

Facet joints allow you to bend forward, bend backward, and twist.

The Dryness In Arthritis

AS YOUR DISCS age and dry out due to water loss, they may lose height, which puts pressure on the facet joints and can result in arthritis. This contributes to the "shrinkage" that happens as we age and lose a few inches in height.

and her lifestyle, that the pain was originating in the facets. She was an avid tennis player, and the pain emerged when she was playing, but improved when she rested.

Irritation in the facet joints causes significant discomfort that can mimic the signs and symptoms of sciatica. This can make the diagnosis of facet pain challenging. One clue to the diagnosis of facet joint pain is how and when it started. Because the facet can be pulled apart or excessively stretched, especially with a strong torquing motion, it tends to affect golfers and tennis players. I've seen a number of world-class tennis players with facet joint pain. The tennis serve, in particular, hyperextends the lower back and stretches the facets. A British study found that the rate of facet joint disease was four to five times higher in tennis players than that of the general population. Recall, too, my own personal story of barely surviving a full-body massage, during which the masseuse moonwalked on my back. An unfortunate side effect of this otherwise wonderful experience was that the masseuse dislocated my facet joint (she likely stretched the nerve-filled capsule around the facet, which accounted for all the pain). My vacation ended and I essentially had to be carted back home as I lay flat on my back. My surgical colleagues were convinced that I had a herniated disc, but it was only after injections of lidocaine and steroids directly into the facet that I finally felt better. This is typically how the diagnosis of facet joint syndrome is confirmed, as an injection of local anesthetic and an anti-inflammatory medication into the affected joints often bring instant and dramatic pain relief.

IS YOUR PAIN COMING FROM A FACET?

SIGNS OF A FACET PAIN GENERATOR: pain or tenderness in the lower back; pain that increases with twisting or arching the body (think of activities such as tennis that involve lots of torquing, or turning); a deep, dull pain that moves to the buttocks or the back of the thighs; stiffness or difficulty with certain movements, such as standing up straight or out of a chair.

COMMON CAUSES: physical trauma/injury; changes associated with aging that cause the cartilaginous cushion that covers the bones to wear away (thus causing pain as the bones of the joint rub together); irritated or pinched nerves that branch out from the spinal nerve and supply the facet joints; poor posture; infection; disc degeneration.

QUESTIONS TO ASK YOURSELF: Do you have to turn your entire body to look over to the right or left? Do you feel pain in other areas, such as your shoulders, mid-back, buttocks, thighs (but not below the knee)? Is your pain one-sided (unilateral)? Is it hard to stand up straight and lift yourself out of a chair? Do you play tennis or golf? Was the onset of pain sudden and upon performing a specific act, such as bending to tie your shoelaces or returning a wicked-fast serve in tennis with your backhand stroke?

If you answered yes to any combination of these questions, then your pain could be originating from a facet joint. The main clue to a facet pain generator is that certain body positions make the pain worse or, conversely, better. Typically, clues to the diagnosis can be found on an MRI or CT scan; alternatively, the diagnosis also can be determined using a therapeutic block whereby a painkiller is injected right into the facet joint and relief is felt almost immediately.

Pain Generator #6: Neural Foramina

The neural (intervertebral) foramen is the opening between every two vertebrae where the nerve roots exit the spine. The nerve roots travel through the foramen to reach the rest of your body. There are two neural foramina between each pair of vertebrae, one on each side. Without the foramen, nerve fibers and the signals they carry could not travel to and from the brain.

Neural foramen stenosis is seen most often in older adults. If you are over fifty, it's likely that your MRI report will include, in addition to the radiologist's description of disc bulges, diminution in disc height, etc., the term *foraminal stenosis*. In general, *stenosis* refers to a narrowing of a passage in the body. Hence, if you have a narrowing of that area of the spine where the nerves leave your spinal canal, it's called neural foraminal stenosis. You can also have spinal stenosis, which typically means you have a narrowing of the canal in the back of the spine through which the spinal cord and nerves travel downward. This canal extends from the top of the cervical spine to your sacrum.

As noted previously, the natural aging process causes our discs to

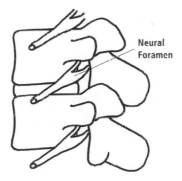

Neural
Foramen

The intervertebral foramen is the opening through which the nerve roots exit the spine and travel to the rest of the body. There are two neural foramina located between each pair of vertebrae, one on each side. The foramen creates a protective passageway for the nerves that carry signals between the spinal cord and the rest of the body.

AS OUR POPULATION gets older, the incidence of spinal stenosis, also known as spinal claudication, becomes more common and with it the problem of foraminal stenosis. Check out how many older folks bend over their shopping carts in the grocery store; not only could these people be suffering from some age-related osteoporosis, but they likely have spinal stenosis, for which flexing forward improves or even relieves their symptoms.

degenerate, thereby decreasing the disc height, and as a direct consequence, narrowing the foramen. Many arthritic conditions narrow the foramina, slowly squeezing the nerves and causing pain and possibly weakness and loss of sensation. Since this is a slow process, it's more common in the elderly or those with existing arthritic conditions. It is also an eminently treatable condition if recognized. If your physician suspects this diagnosis, he or she will need to order the proper imaging studies.

Coming up, we'll review all the treatment options for the Six Pain Generators. Sometimes, as is the case with treating spinal stenosis, the options may be controversial—much more so than making the diagnosis. I'll discuss many of the issues and present my ideas of potentially effective treatments in order from least to most invasive. In the next step, however, we'll take a short detour to discuss the ways in which you can gather your information and present it to your doctor.

ACTION PLAN

- Make sure you have a general understanding of the Six Pain Generators: muscles, soft tissues, bones, discs, facets, and neural foramina.
- Go through each and every set of questions in this chapter. Even though you may believe you've got a problem with a disc, it helps

IS YOUR PAIN COMING FROM A NEURAL FORAMEN?

SIGNS OF A NEURAL FORAMEN PAIN GENERATOR: chronic nerve pain that didn't come on suddenly—it's gradual and feels like a gnawing, dull pain rather than one that is sharp; back pain and especially leg pain or cramping that gets worse with walking and improves with rest and bending forward (and the pulses in the legs are strong, so there's no vascular issues).

COMMON CAUSES: arthritis, advanced age.

QUESTIONS TO ASK YOURSELF: Are you over the age of fifty-five? Do you have a family history of osteoarthritis, rheumatoid arthritis, or psoriatic arthritis?

If you answered yes to any of these questions, then your pain could be originating from a neural foramen. A common first test to confirm the diagnosis is with an X-ray, because you can see the foramen on the scan; additionally, it often helps to inject lidocaine and a steroid into the foramen to see if the pain subsides. (More on this in chapter 7.)

to have a big-picture view of your back's health. The sets of questions in this chapter will provide you with lots of clues to consider in moving forward and approaching a doctor for help. I've hinted at some of the methods used to diagnose many of the conditions associated with these pain generators. I'll be going into much greater detail in upcoming chapters. For now, look back at your responses, modify any of the answers you gave in the checklist on pages 4–6, and get ready to take your second step.

Step 2

Prepare to Work with
Health Care Professionals

AS A CHILD I FELL IN LOVE WITH PUZZLES AND BRAINTEASERS. I watched Charlie Chan and read Sherlock Holmes novels. I can vividly recall how disappointed I became if I didn't pick up the clues to solve the mystery before the TV program or the book ended.

Physicians, regardless of their specialty, need to be good diagnosticians; they need to read the clues and solve the diagnostic puzzle. Even today, I don't look at any patient's MRI or CT scan before I've taken a complete history and examined him or her in person. I want to make a clear diagnosis based on the clues and not on the pictures. And I certainly don't want to see the imaging results first and then have the patient's history or my physical findings "fit" the pictures. This is important, because if the MRI, CT scans, or other imaging test doesn't match my clinical diagnosis and impression, I need to rethink the entire problem.

When Dr. Jerome Groopman's best-selling book *How Doctors Think* came out a few years ago, it provided much-needed insights into the mind of the physician and how the layperson could best capitalize on this perspective to be a better-educated patient (and, therefore, an active participant in the treatment of his or her medical issues). In a similar vein, the goal of this step is to equip you with an arsenal of information that will help you deliver the right kind of information to your doctor in order to seek the right diagnosis.

In the last step, I gave you a comprehensive tour of the Six Pain Generators and how certain symptoms reflect different pain generators. You may already have a vague idea as to what's causing your pain, or you may have enough information to initiate a conversation with your doctor. I'll warn you, however, that the sleuthing has likely just begun. Far too often, patients visit their doctors, thinking that it's solely the doctor's responsibility to magically solve the problem. Patients assume that somehow their doctor already knows what's wrong and what treatment should follow. Many also believe that an MRI will show exactly what's wrong. But this couldn't be further from the truth. This part explores the common challenges doctors face in searching for the treatment that is right for you and why the key to arriving at an accurate diagnosis will continue to rest within you, the patient. I'm going to force you to go much deeper than the previous step in creating an atlas of all symptoms. The goal is to become a staunch advocate for yourself when dealing with health care professionals and working with them as a team.

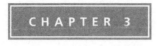

CHAPTER 3

How to Be a Staunch
Advocate for Yourself

G ETTING A HANDLE ON your symptoms is one thing, but conveying them to your health care providers and moving to that next step in dealing with your symptoms is another. Just as my wife can't definitively know what I want for my birthday without my specifically telling her, a doctor will know only as much about your medical history as you're willing to verbalize or reveal. There is no oracle for back pain when you show up for a "reading." Again, I reiterate that initially, your diagnosis relies more on what *you* have to offer than what your doctor does.

Unfortunately, doctors frequently don't give their patients the attention they deserve. Even when there is a straightforward medical problem such as a blocked artery, inguinal hernia, or arthritis, many doctors would rather skip long-winded explanations, preferring instead to deal with the problem as expeditiously as possible and move on to the next patient. Much of this has to do with the economics of twenty-first-century medicine. The reality is that the modern medical paradigm is leading more and more physicians to spend less and less time with patients. Moreover, many physicians who treat low back pain as part of their busy general practice are not sufficiently familiar with or particularly interested in the detailed anatomy of the back. They appreciate that in most cases low back pain will heal itself regardless of the treatment suggested, so they skip to the bottom line: How do I treat the pain as quickly as possible?

This problem is further compounded when there's no precise diagnosis or identifiable pain generator, which is the case in many instances of low back pain. But chances are you're reading this book because you have ongoing back pain and suffer from chronic relapses. Without an accurate diagnosis, your doctor must carefully review symptoms and complaints—a much more laborious endeavor. And a doctor who can't identify the source or find any evidence of injury or disease certainly is unlikely to sit down for a chat about spinal anatomy. This is regrettable, since patients can really help themselves by knowing more about their back, how it works, and what can go wrong.

Admittedly, the tendency that I and many other well-intentioned physicians have—the trap that we fall into—is to control the interview in a direction that confirms the diagnosis we've grown accustomed to making based on a few bits of information. So, if I think your back pain is related to your marathon running, I'll find a way to confirm that through the types of questions I ask. Does it hurt after you run? Do you stretch? Have you considered better running shoes? (Which, by the way, may be the most common cause of back pain in runners!) We essentially try to "lead the witness" so that we gather further information that fits neatly into one or another of our diagnostic boxes. But this can lead us astray, because we can become far too interested in turning off our ears and interrupting the patient with questions. Doctors interrupt their patients within eighteen seconds, on average, of the start of their conversation. I was no less guilty of this recently, when I met a patient referred to me for a "herniated disc."

The Bus Driver Who Taught Me to Be a Better Listener

Mr. B was not unlike many other patients referred by their primary doctors: He had experienced, according to his internist, severe pain in his lower back and particularly in his legs. His physician had started an entire course of conservative treatment, including the usual regimen of analgesics and muscle relaxants. When his symptoms didn't improve, his physician ordered an MRI, which revealed a disc bulge, and so he ended up in my office.

In taking his medical history, I learned that Mr. B was a fifty-four-year-old right-handed father of three mostly grown children. He drove a bus in New York City, and he played the part well—as straightforward and crotchety as anyone who's lived his whole life in New York. But he was also tough, so tough that I imagined he tolerated pain pretty well. He lived in the Bronx and was eligible for a pension but was so well motivated that he opted not to take it. Like I said, this man was very resilient . . . until his back made him less so, and he needed to do something about it.

Patients like this really fascinate me. I admire those who forgo a pension because they are so devoted to their work that they prefer to continue onward as always. Before I met him in person, his information on record revealed a lot to me, enough to feel that this was someone I could really help. His past medical history was significant for the fact that he was overweight, which was not surprising, since he sat in a bus eight hours a day. He was also slightly hypertensive and took medication to address that, in addition to his high cholesterol. When I conducted my physical exam, I began my usual routine of asking questions about his pain: Where is it? How long have you had pain? When does your pain get worse or better? I must have used the word *pain* in every single question, and in doing so had totally missed the one word he kept replying with: *cramps*. I kept referring to his pain—not appreciating that cramps, rather than classic pain, were his issue.

Mr. B had already done his homework; he'd educated himself on spinal anatomy and the symptoms of low back pain. As I kept referring to his leg pain, he finally said, "Doc, you're not listening to me. I don't have *pain*. I have bad leg *cramps*!" His response was startling; he shook me out of the trancelike state that most physicians enter when going through the motions of asking questions. Indeed, I was caught red-handed—I was trying to fit my diagnosis into the box that had come with the referral from his primary doctor (who had assumed it was a herniated disc). Mr. B forced me to stop and listen with different ears, and it immediately occurred to me that he was taking Lipitor to control his cholesterol. I knew that one of this statin's side effects is severe leg cramping. We switched him to a different statin he could take without such side effects, and the "pain" went away. In this instance, Mr. B appreciated his symptoms more accurately than I did.

I suspect that Mr. B's internist was a bit embarrassed that he hadn't figured that out himself, but both of us learned a lot from this intrepid man. For one, it's important to be your own advocate. Had this man not given himself a small lesson on biological jargon, he might not have known to use the word *cramp* instead of *pain*. We also learned an invaluable lesson about perception: It's critical for doctors not to pigeonhole their thinking processes, though I suppose it's human to do so. And third, this case proved the power of looking at all of the clues that might be causing a symptom. On the surface, a cholesterol-lowering drug, especially one as popular as Lipitor, wouldn't seem to have anything to do with back pain, or pain in general, for that matter. But therein lies proof to the complexity of the human body.

I chide myself for exhibiting some of the same behaviors I observe—and am critical of—in my colleagues. Why do so many of us fall into this trap? It's because we physicians are trained to congregate signs and symptoms together to make a diagnosis. We are conditioned to affix symptoms, even when they are complicated or don't seem to make sense, to certain diagnoses. And we can often miss important symptoms, which then lead us down the wrong pathways to the wrong diagnosis. Once again, we have the twin powers of time and human error working against us. The exigencies of medical practice limit the time we spend with patients, so we hear less. We also tend to hear what we want to hear (i.e., those symptoms that fit neatly with our diagnosis) and subconsciously disregard what doesn't fit. Ironically, *the parts that don't fit may be the key to the diagnosis!*

Patients like Mr. B are few and far between. I'm not referring to this man's long and, no doubt, frustrating wait to obtain an accurate diagnosis; I'm talking about the manner in which he showed up in my office. He had done some research. He had taken the time to look up words to describe his condition and his uncomfortable sensations. He was, put simply, the ideal patient. That's what you can become, using the guidelines and worksheets in this chapter.

I realize that every doctor works differently. In writing this next section so that it will be most useful to you, I decided first to share how I approach new patients when they first come to visit me in my office. If you see things from my perspective, it can help you immensely with optimizing your visit with your own doctor. This will help you know what's probably going on in your doctor's head as he or she examines you and tries to understand your history as well as your current pain.

Taking Your History

Sometimes taking a patient's history begins before I've even set my eyes on them. It can start as a comment that the patient makes to my staff when he or she calls to make the appointment. Luckily, my staff is trained to take extra time with patients in order to make them feel comfortable and to answer their questions. Through this process, my staff frequently acquires an initial "feel" for people and can begin the process of cluing me in to what I'm about to encounter. Is the patient anxious? If so, why? Does the patient fear that surgery may be needed? Or is that anxiety related to more mundane issues, such as dealing with their insurance? Or perhaps the patient is in a great deal of pain and needs to be seen earlier than the next available appointment.

Patients who come across as rude and demanding to my staff can also clue me in to their fears, allowing me to better handle their concerns in a constructive way. Next to the general observations made by my staff, the patients' gait as my staff escorts them from the waiting room to the examination room can be quite informative. I'll watch from a distance and pick up further clues to the problem. Do they favor one side when they walk? Are they standing straight up? Are they dragging their feet? Do they need an assisted device to walk?

One of my professors, the great Columbia neurologist Dr. Daniel Sciarra, had us imitate the various neurological gaits. It was an invaluable exercise for us in training. The gait of someone with sciatica is very different from that of someone with peripheral neuropathy, Parkinson's disease, or one who has suffered a stroke.

My mentors lived in an age before sophisticated imaging. They relied almost exclusively on teasing out the nuances and subtleties from the history and physical. This is an art that is being rapidly lost, because it is so much easier to just look at the images. My professors, men like Dr. Carmen Vicale, also taught me the importance of the relationship that needs to be established between doctor and patient. I remember clearly how often they would hold patients' hands or quietly put their arms around them.

In many offices, the history and even the physical exam are now performed by physician extenders—physician assistants, nurse practitioners, or interns and residents who may be fully competent at what they do—but the information they convey to the treating physician (the person who the patients have actually come to see) is now second-hand. What's missing in the process could very well be the most critical ingredient to the patient-doctor relationship: face-to-face time, time for us to get to know each other, the time to build trust and confidence, a time to get a glimpse at the character of your physician, and an opportunity for me to glimpse into your life beyond your "chief complaint." I can't speak for every doctor out there, but it helps that I really like people and love what I do.

I feel my first responsibility to all new patients is to ease their anxiety and gain their confidence. I make it a habit to introduce myself without the doctor prefix and try to find some commonality with patients. It may relate to where they live, what they do, or anything that is open and honest and breaks the ice. Once I do this, which really takes only a few short minutes, my next task is to listen. Just listen.

Once I've established a rapport with patients, I review what's called the intake form with them and ensure that nothing was excluded. This form chronicles a patient's history and summarizes the main details of that person's health. It's critical that you, as the patient, come as prepared as possible to fill out this form. And it can be extensive, asking many questions about your health history and that of your family. It will even ask questions that seem remotely related to back pain, such as a possible history of cancer or diabetes. It's amazing how much people omit because they don't think it's important. These questionnaires are mailed to my patients prior to their first visit with me, and they are instructed to fill them out as completely as they can before stepping into my office. I hope your physician has a similar practice, and I encourage you to be as thorough and honest as you can. In addition to asking the usual questions about your name, age, marital status, and so on, the intake form will also ask for a slew of information that can be helpful in getting to know you—and your back. This includes your height and weight; whether you're right- or

COLLAGEN VASCULAR DISEASES: Collagen is a tough, glue-like protein that makes up 30 percent of body protein. It shapes the structure of tendons, bones, and connective tissues. Problems with the immune system can affect these structures, which can then lead to back pain. Collagen vascular diseases include dermatomyositis, polyarteritis nodosa, rheumatoid arthritis, scleroderma, and systemic lupus erythematosus.

left-handed; your history of tobacco, drug, and alcohol use; prescribed medications, with a reminder not to forget to list vitamins and supplements; previous surgeries or procedures and the dates they were performed; allergies; etc. You'll be asked about a potential family history of osteo-, rheumatoid, psoriatic, or other arthritic conditions, and lupus or other collagen vascular diseases. Come with knowledge about whether or not any family members have had spinal surgery, chiropractic care, pain management, and the like.

I'll then review the intake form with you, line by line, to finish taking your history. Before I proceed with an examination, there is always one question that I ask: "Is there anything we did not discuss that you think I need to know?"

This accomplishes two things. For one, it gives patients another opportunity to contribute information that they feel may be useful, particularly at that moment when, hopefully, some trust has been established and issues that are below the surface can be discussed. Second, it affirms the feeling that they are not rushed and that I am here to listen further.

It must be reiterated: Being prepared before you see your doctor will make the time spent with your physician much more productive. It will give you an opportunity to think about your problem in the quiet of your home, and give you the opportunity to review your problem with those around you, who almost always have something to contribute that you do not see or appreciate. Organizing and preparing a record of, well, you, are so vital to reaching an accurate diagnosis that I've re-created a version of my own intake sheet on page 64 that you can use to get ahead of yourself.

Prepare a Timeline and a Record

It pays to be well versed in your history so that you can communicate your facts concisely. Start by creating a timeline of your back pain— when it started, why you think it started, and any relevant information to include. It also helps to gather all the information you can about your medical history and organize it in a single location, such as a notebook. For those who are tech-savvy, create a document that you can file away on your computer, or better yet, upload a file to an Internet-based cloud, which you can access on your phone, so that when your doctor asks for certain information, it's all there for you to refer to.

At the beginning of Step 1, I gave you a checklist to fill out. Now let's go a bit further and list additional items of import (again, I recommend answering these questions to their fullest and being as thorough and honest as you can; use a notebook or create a document on your computer using Word or Excel, or alternatively, go online to www.drjackstern.com and download a version of this worksheet). Even though your doctor or any specialist you see will have you fill out similar forms, having a "rough draft" will be of enormous help. What's more, if your doctor's office doesn't ask for any of the information below, you can provide it as an addition to create a more comprehensive picture of you and your pain. The investigative work starts at home. Use the following worksheet to think about and write down lifestyle factors that could be contributing to your back pain.

- Approximate dates of onset of the symptoms:

  _____

- Are the symptoms related to an event, such as a car accident, work accident, accident at home, or something else? Did they occur during (circle all that apply): lifting, pulling, pushing, twisting, falling, bending, reaching, squatting?
- Were you hit by an object?   Yes/No
- Approximate dates of when the symptoms may have changed and circumstances under which they have changed:

  _____

- Approximate dates of all previous treatments for your low back pain, who performed the treatments, any notes from the treating physicians as to how the treatment was done, and your response to the treatment:

  _____
  _____
  _____

- What makes your pain feel better?

  _____

- What makes your pain feel worse?

  _____

- A list of all previous surgeries, even if you think they have no particular relationship to your low back pain.
- Copies of all your imaging studies and the radiologist report.
- Family history, especially as it pertains to arthritic conditions and low back pain.

List all drugs (over-the-counter and prescription) that you take:

_____

List all supplements and vitamins that you take:

_____

List all sports that you play, including hobbies and activities that get your body moving:

_____

What do you do for a living?

_____

What are your main job-related tasks?

_____

What *physical* tasks are involved in your job (e.g., typing, lifting,
  pulling, bending, reaching, pushing, twisting, squatting, sitting)? List all that apply.

_____

**Are You Currently Having Problems
with Any of the Following:**

Yes/No	Describe all Yes responses
Eyes	
Ears, nose, throat	
Lungs, breathing	
Heart	
Digestion	
Bowel movement	
Bladder problems	
Diabetes	
High blood pressure	
Bleeding	
Numbness/tingling	
Blackout/fainting	
Psychological problems	
AIDS	
Cancer	
Arthritis	
Polio	
TB	
Headaches	

There are two sets of questions that I ask patients, and on the surface these questions may not seem to have anything to do with back pain. But they can have everything to do with back pain. Be prepared for them:

- *How is your job?* Is it stressful? Does it cause back pain? If your job doesn't involve any back-related movement or obvious signs of back pain–related triggers, I would then move on to ask about your hobbies or sports. Which activities cause back pain? Does gardening or tennis affect how you feel? What about the things that make your back pain better? I ask patients to discuss their activities and what positions cause pain and what positions alleviate pain.

- *Do you have any difficulty controlling your bowels or your bladder, or have you noticed any change in sexual function?* The answer to this final set of questions can be particularly insightful, especially in a patient who is experiencing any loss of strength or sensation. I'll discuss what this can mean at greater length when I review the warning signs of a serious neurological condition.

If your doctor doesn't ask versions of these questions, offer the answers anyway. When in doubt, volunteer the information, even if you don't think it's remotely related to your back. And to illustrate the significance of this, I want you to meet Lucy. Her story provides a good case in point:

I immediately recognized the warning signs when I took inventory of Lucy's history and the number of imaging tests she had already undergone. When the X-rays, CT scans, and MRIs are so numerous that their very weight gives me low back pain, then I know I'm in for a challenge! Lucy's file was no exception. I gave her credit, though, for letting her husband, Steve, accompany her to see me. I frequently find the clues to a patient's back problem in the person who shows up to be their advocate. And again, Lucy's case was no exception in this regard. Steve sat in a chair armed with a pen and notepad. Noticing how poised they both were, I quickly got the sense that they were well-educated professionals who'd done as much homework as they could.

Unlike patients whose weight can be a factor in their back pain, Lucy occupied the other end of the spectrum. She was a thin 115 pounds on a five-foot-seven-inch frame. The couple had three school-aged daughters, so I inferred that their lives were busy. Lucy also worked part-time as a publicist for a small business. And when I asked Lucy to describe herself, she said passionately, "I'm a runner." Due to the back pain, running hadn't been on her agenda lately, but I understood what she meant. I typically find that runners take ownership of their sport with a spirited force; once a runner, always a runner. So, for Lucy to make this declaration at a time when running was out of the question for her, I took that to be a loud cry for help. Lucy could not feel like herself or gain any sense of normalcy in her life as she stood on the sidelines.

It was clear that she'd been to at least a half-dozen other physicians, none of whom helped ease her pain. And every conceivable imaging study had been done, none of which yielded a diagnosis. Lucy and Steve were frustrated and anxious, and rightfully so. They had their guard up when I met them, but I probably wouldn't have trusted me, either, if I were in their shoes. To them, I was just another doctor who would probably fail the test. There is an expression in medicine that "the last doctor [i.e., the one who finally makes the diagnosis] is the smartest," but I didn't think that distinction was going to be mine.

For the previous two years, Lucy had developed progressive low back pain, though it didn't radiate down her legs. The pain was constant, and worsened with activity. I watched Lucy sit slumped over and looking uncomfortable. One would think her imaging studies would have turned up something, but all of them were remarkably normal. Lucy also passed her physical exam with flying colors except for a few "mechanical signs." That is, she had pain when I asked her to bend forward or bend backward. But the pain was relatively nonspecific—she couldn't pinpoint the exact spot from where the pain originated. It just hurt everywhere in her lower back, a dull and gnawing pain.

I could easily have gone in circles ruminating over what little clues I had. But then I asked a single question that changed everything: "How is the pain affecting your life and your family?" Her husband seized control of the conversation right away, and Pandora's box was fully open.

No sooner did I pose this question than it became very evident that Lucy was under tremendous stress—a stress that affected her whole family. She had not been eating properly and had toned down her exercising regimen to nearly nothing. Fortunately, her husband offered up this information in a kind and empathetic way, such that Lucy could appreciate his concerns and begin to acknowledge the volume of stress she was under. I don't think she was surprised when I suggested that her treatment would have little to do with her back per se, and that it was time to connect her with a nutritionist, personal trainer, and a meditation class. No doctor had yet to recommend these ideas, which probably encouraged Lucy to be receptive to them because they were "new." She had nothing to lose and a pain-free back to gain.

Four months later, Lucy's pain had all but vanished and she was preparing for another marathon. Had she expressed resistance to the concept that most of her pain was stress-related, she might not have been willing to take the active steps to heal.

ONE THING IS for sure: All of this is just a reminder of how many variables make up our pain equations, especially those that contribute to that expansive space we call the back and which we use every day. It's also a reminder that in addition to the science of medicine, there is still the art of medicine. Sometimes we can't even begin to understand the complexity of the human body and the myriad ways in which it can experience harm and translate that to pain.

Clearly my ability to help this woman came from a combination of experience and the lessons learned from my teachers to listen and to commit to gathering as much information as I possibly can about the problem. It's humbling to consider how many times I have missed the diagnosis and the effects my own failures have had on other people's lives.

So, with that in mind, let's turn to the physical exam. Once your foundation is established through your history and record of past medical exams or procedures, the next step is to learn more from a current physical exam.

Physical Examination

The components of physical exams tend to be pretty standard. Make sure your physician has examined you for the following:

1. *Gait:* How do you walk? Your gait gives important clues to your diagnosis.
2. *Spinal mobility:* Which positions are painful and which are not? This simple piece of information can direct your doctor to make a specific diagnosis, as certain pain generators cause pain when you're in a specific position, and the pain subsides when you're not in that position.
3. *Inspection of the muscle groups:* Does your doctor find any signs of atrophy and fasciculations? Atrophy would refer to loss of muscle

mass and strength. Fasciculations are small, involuntary muscle twitches.

4. *Strength:* What's the difference between your dominant and non-dominant side? Your doctor can perform a test to compare. This is one reason why my intake form asks whether you are right- or left-handed. This information isn't always so black-and-white, as some individuals are ambidextrous; they typically use one particular hand but can just as easily use the other. And then there are a smaller number of patients who may be right- or left-handed, but the opposite leg is their dominant one. So, they would normally write with their right hand but kick a ball with their left foot. Such information is important because if I know only that they are right-handed, but their right foot seems slightly weaker, it may not be a sign of a neurological problem, but rather that they are left-foot dominant.

5. *Sensory testing:* How do you respond to various stimuli, such as a pinprick, vibrations, changes in position, and perceptions of hot and cold? These can give subtle but important clues. A patient with a herniated disc, for example, may normally have a great deal of pain, but may also have a problem telling me where I'm poking him and where he feels the vibration of a tuning fork that I've applied to his skin. On the other hand, a patient with misfiring neurons somewhere frequently has a combination of sensory loss (he cannot identify my probing) and dull, gnawing pain.

6. *Reflexes:* What are your reflexes like? Are they strong, weak, exaggerated, or is there an asymmetry in how your reflexes respond (e.g., your right knee-jerk reaction is normal, but it's slower on the left side)? Most reflexes are quite complex, requiring a number of synapses in a number of different nuclei in the central nervous system. So, a quick check of your reflexes is a very rough test of your nervous system's functionality and may give a clue to which specific nerves are involved in your particular problem.

Once your doctor has finished examining you, hopefully you and your doctor can develop some sense of the source of your pain.

Should You Get an X-Ray and/or MRI Right Away?

Is imaging always necessary? Interestingly, there really is no universal standard for imaging back pain. These are the current absolute reasons for getting an X-ray, and the vast majority of people who have back pain don't fall into any of these categories: (1) history of recent trauma, such as a car accident or fall, (2) unexplained weight loss, (3) unexplained fever, (4) immunosuppression, or a compromised immune system due to medications or illness, (5) history of cancer, (6) history of intravenous drug use, (7) history of prolonged corticosteroid use, (8) osteoporosis, and (9) over the age of seventy years.

Even in the absence of these reasons, many physicians will not hesitate to order expensive and occasionally invasive imaging tests. For most patients, no imaging test is needed. Imaging tests are frequently an adjunct to diagnosing spinal problems. And in many cases

Read, Look, Listen

IMAGING ISN'T ALWAYS the best way to diagnose. Reading a patient's medical history on record, including current questionnaires, looking at a patient and performing various tests in person, and listening to his or her stories and what's conveyed within the confines of an intimate exam room can do more for arriving at an accurate diagnosis—and proper treatment—than anything else. Which then brings up an important lesson: Patients need to support their doctors in the task of reading, looking, and listening.

of back pain, current imaging technology will not detect what is really wrong with someone. A thorough medical history, complete physical exam, and an attentive ear are the cornerstones for identifying a majority of the causes of back pain.

Like a good detective, your doctor needs to collect all of the data about you and your back pain and make sense of it. What makes this somewhat easier is that most causes of low back pain originate from only a relatively small number of distinct sources. As we saw in the previous chapter, these are referred to as the pain generators. Needless to say, I cannot discuss every potential cause of patients' pain, and it's for this reason that we have an adage in medicine that "common diseases occur commonly." It means that, as trained doctors and diagnosticians, we have learned to always first consider the most likely clinical explanation for a patient's situation before considering "zebras," or uncommon, rare explanations.

By now you should have a good foundation for understanding your spinal anatomy and possibly even the source of your pain. Now let's turn to the heart of the matter: potential solutions. In Step 3, I'm going to explore what a physician like me starts to think about when someone like you enters my office, and what you can do to support healing based on possible diagnoses. A prominent theme will run throughout the rest of the book: The goal is less about finding the magic bullet than it is about avoiding the slippery slope of being a patient who has a single episode of back pain to becoming a patient with lifelong chronic pain. If you can find relief through tactical strategies and learn how to manage your pain so that it doesn't interrupt your life and ability to do the things you want to do, then you'll feel that you have succeeded.

ACTION PLAN

• To find an excellent doctor, you'll need to do two things: Start with your primary-care physician, and ask around your circle of trusted friends and colleagues for referrals. You'll likely need to start with your primary-care doctor for insurance purposes, and sometimes that's the only person you need to find relief.

- Before setting foot through any doctor's door, make sure that you've got your medical history down pat, including the history of close family members (siblings, parents, and grandparents). Use the worksheets in this chapter to organize and gather the information you need to present to a doctor.

- Conduct your own mini self-exam while in the comfort of home and bring your results with you to your doctor. This will help you to maximize every minute you have with your doctor.

- Even though you may not think that certain medications, vitamins, and supplements have anything to do with your back, list them out and show them to your doctor. The same goes for other medical conditions that you may have been treated for in the past or are currently managing (e.g., diabetes, high cholesterol, cancer, an old sports injury). Be honest about your lifestyle habits, too. Do you smoke or drink? Train for triathlons?

- Don't be alarmed if imaging tests are not ordered right away. If your symptoms don't fall into certain categories, then your best solution may be to avoid imaging for now and commence a treatment plan attuned to your specific symptoms.

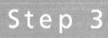
Step 3

Ensure Proper Diagnosis

I REALIZE THAT MANY OF YOU READING THIS BOOK ARE NOT DEAL-ing with your first episode of back pain. You may very well be among the millions who are managing the pain on an ongoing basis. In 2007, the American College of Physicians and the American Pain Society divided back pain patients into three broad categories, two of which associate back pain with a specific cause, such as spinal stenosis or a fractured vertebra. The term they opted to use to describe the third category, which probably best describes your clinical situation, is "nonspecific low back pain." This, in layman's language, pretty much means "I don't know exactly what's causing your back pain."

I believe this category is poorly named, because "nonspecific" leads the health care provider and the patient to feel that there is no "specific" treatment. But in my experience, there is a wide assortment of effective treatments available. Admittedly, this can involve trying several treatments in succession until you find the one that works for you, and it may even require a combination of treatments. Indeed, this process is typically one of trial and failure, and I will venture that some of you have already been down that path.

I've given you a lot of information to absorb and homework to do in hopes that you can begin to understand your particular type and cause of back pain. But what I haven't done yet, and what this giant step sets forth to achieve, is guide you through the thought process that a physician like me undertakes when presented with a patient like you. Once you have an appreciation for my train of thought, then, as part of the same big step, I'll take you through the common treatment options that are linked to certain (known) causes of back pain, what we've been referring to as the pain generators. The point of this exercise is to show you the serendipity involved in finding back pain relief, and to demonstrate the complexity of the often tedious approach to diagnosing and treating back pain. It's also in hopes that you secure a proper diagnosis.

CHAPTER 4

How a Doctor Like Me Thinks About the Challenge of Low Back Pain

THE STATISTICS REGARDING LOW back pain can create some initial bias for medical providers. Of all cases of mechanical low back pain, a whopping 70 percent are due to lumbar strain or sprain, which typically heals itself over time, usually within six weeks. Ten percent are caused by age-related degenerative changes to the discs and facets; a scant 4 percent are due to herniated discs; another 4 percent are due to osteoporotic compression fractures; and only a mere 3 percent are due to spinal stenosis. All other causes account for less than 1 percent of cases.

What these statistics tell me is that most of you have low back pain as a result of muscular or soft tissue injury. Your pain is localized to the area of the low back; it doesn't shoot down your leg, radiate higher up your back, or around to your belly or chest. This is important to remember, as the *site* of your pain is a clue to the source of your pain. Other key facts, which I emphasized earlier, but serve as a good reminder, include:

- Does your pain *spread* very far? To other areas of your body?
- What are the *quality* and *intensity* of your pain?
- How would you describe your pain's frequency and duration? How often does the pain come on and how long does it last?

Most patients with low back pain will describe the quality of the pain as an ache or spasm. On a scale of 1 to 10, it averages at 5 to 6. It is rarely so severe that it requires a trip to the emergency room or the need for narcotics. Patients also will relate that the pain has plagued them for several years, and that with every ensuing year the episodes of low back pain become more frequent and the duration of the episodes much longer. Many patients will also notice local tenderness and that their mobility has become more and more limited.

I find it interesting that when pressed to remember, a large number of my patients do recall the worst episode of pain and how it began. It's usually some traumatic event, or sometimes a relatively minor one, such as slipping on the sidewalk or falling while reaching for an object. The typical scenario is one in which the individual engaged in an activity that was beyond the ability of his muscular and soft tissue structures to absorb. I like referring to these patients as "weekend warriors." They are inadequately fit to perform the activity, which can be any number of things such as shoveling the entire driveway after a snowfall, spending the whole day working in the garden, or shooting thirty-six holes of golf when nine or eighteen would have been much more sensible. The most common modes of onset involve sports-related injury, lifting injury, pain that began with an accident at work, pain as a result of an automobile accident, and, for women, childbirth. My patients will also describe the things that make the pain worse and those that make it better. They might also know what

THE RED FLAGS are signs or symptoms that might indicate an infection, spinal tumor, fracture, or serious neurological disease. These include: fever; trouble with speech, motor skills, muscle actions, coordination, balance, and vision; abnormal reflexes; loss of sensation; inability to walk correctly; and inability to control bladder and bowels.

medications help alleviate the pain. All this information gives me clues to the source of their pain.

But let's take a step back for a moment so I can share what's going through my mind when a patient first enters my office. The statistics tell one story, but it's my job to help flesh that story out and make it consistent with your unique situation and set of circumstances. Let's say you're a new patient who has come to see me with a chief complaint of low back pain, and you don't necessarily know if or when the "accident" happened to cause your pain. It would seem that my first task would be to come up with a diagnosis, but in fact this is not my top priority during your initial visit. My first concern is excluding the diagnosis you *don't* have and particularly those conditions that may be life-threatening or a harbinger of serious neurological problems. Many of my patients don't verbalize the fear that their back pain is actually an indication of a more serious condition. As a doctor, it's actually comforting to know that your pain has been there for a while and that it's confined to the low back. This tends to eliminate those serious, acute diseases. Your pain may originate elsewhere in your body, but the fact that you don't have what's called a neurological deficit probably eliminates an emergency situation. By definition, a neurological deficit is a functional abnormality due to a decrease in the function of the brain, spinal cord, muscles, or nerves. Common examples include the inability to speak, loss of sensation, loss of balance, abnormal reflexes, walking problems, and the inability to control your bladder and bowels. Once I've ruled out the serious diagnoses, I then have the luxury of time—time to spend with you and continue to search for the source of your pain.

On the other end of the spectrum, if you come to me with an avatar that has X's and Y's covering both sides of the body and extending down to the leg and up the back and even the cervical spine, I know from experience that helping you will be extraordinarily difficult. Widespread symptoms of long-standing duration that have failed a multitude of conventional and sometimes unconventional treatments are difficult to treat, and it's unlikely that I will be successful. I want to reiterate that this doesn't mean that you don't have real pain. You may in fact have real pain, but it probably means that the pain generator may be rooted in the brain or another place, as I will discuss in detail later on.

The First Line of Action

Common diagnoses are common, so let's assume that you're like the patient I first described, with classic, typical low back pain. I can make several more assumptions about your medical care to date. I'll assume that your physician has ordered and reviewed plain X-rays of your lumbar spine. I'll also venture that these studies—particularly if you are fifty years of age or younger—were normal. The reason I say this is because more than 95 percent of patients with low back pain have normal X-rays, as very few of the known pain generators show abnormalities on X-rays. In fact, muscle, soft tissue, and ligaments are not visible at all on X-rays; X-rays are best for demonstrating bony structures. This also explains why X-rays may be appropriate when low back pain is related to trauma, to rule out broken bones or compression fractures, especially in patients with osteoporosis. They may also be helpful in patients with known cancer, to rule out metastatic disease to bone.

Routine X-rays may also give some indication of discogenic disease if the distance between the vertebrae is diminished. Although they are unusual, other clues on the X-rays can point to problems with the sacroiliac (SI) joint, which is the main joint in the pelvis that supports the spine. This is especially true for older patients who have abnormally large osteoarthritic facet joints. But with the exception of these unusual circumstances, X-rays in general play a minor role in diagnosing the origins of low back pain. This may be a surprise to many of you, but there is no evidence that routine X-rays in patients with nonspecific low back pain are associated with greater improvement in patient outcomes. What's more, exposure to unnecessary radiation should be avoided, particularly in young women.

Nonetheless, if your back pain persists, it's likely that you'll be subjected to a series of lumbar X-rays. Although many physicians will wait two months before ordering X-rays, some will order them sooner because they fear that you may be one of those patients with a more serious condition. And some physicians will request X-rays as a preemptive strike—for fear that a delay in diagnoses could result in further complications that end in a lawsuit. This is just one reason that established protocols are so important. "Preventive medicine" sometimes means preventing a lawsuit, but it also means that a large number of patients are radiated unnecessarily.

If your X-rays come back as normal, most doctors, myself included, will offer the following recommendations to start:

- Rest and avoid painful positions (modification of activities).
- Ice the lower back to relieve the spasm.
- Take non-steroidal anti-inflammatories (e.g., aspirin, ibuprofen, or one of the COX-2 inhibitors, such as Celebrex, which block enzymes responsible for inflammation and pain).
- Try muscle relaxants. The ones I find most effective are carisoprodol (Soma), cyclobenzaprine (Flexeril), and methocarbamol (Robaxin). When the spasms are severe, I prescribe diazepam (Valium).
- Consider weight loss, if appropriate.

- Engage in back-strengthening exercises or a course of physical therapy.

Don't underestimate the power of physical therapy. Like the vast majority of physicians who refer patients for physical therapy, I write a prescription with the diagnosis, give some history, and detail what I hope the therapy will achieve. But I don't specify exactly how I want physical therapists to work with patients. I trust that they are trained and licensed professionals who can choose and even modify the modalities as they see fit. They might decide to use hot packs, cold packs, massage, electrical stimulation, a specific exercise program, stretching and a range of motion exercises, or a combination of any of these as well as others. This diverse approach is one reason why a recent review of more than 1,800 studies (reported in a 2012 issue of *Spine*) showed that there is not a good study validating the effects of a single "best combination" of practices for addressing back pain in everyone. And in another study published that same year, a group of researchers found that exercise—an important component of physical therapy— promotes cell proliferation in different areas of the intervertebral disc and recruits cells that are active in disc regeneration. So, as counterintuitive as it may sound, and as I hinted at earlier, some of the strongest evidence supports treating back pain with exercise, including stretching and some aerobic activity. So keep moving!

REMEMBER, all of these above-mentioned ideas are suggestions to get you through the acute phases of back pain. Most of you will respond to one or more of these treatments and the story ends there; even if the symptoms recur, the treatments are usually again effective. I prescribe the same regimen in my patients for subsequent episodes. But what happens if these treatments are ineffective and symptoms last more than one or two months? At this point, you're experiencing back pain that is present most of the time and you notice that you're irritable, tired, and less energetic than usual. The pain is interfering with your life; you cannot easily get up from your desk at work throughout the day, lift the children, or tend to groceries. It's all too painful. You avoid sports, travel, and sexual activity.

The only exception to the patient whose back is quickly becoming a chronic problem is the person whose posture or a repetitive yet seemingly innocuous activity is to blame, and you might also be surprised by how often this is the case. If you fall into this category, then you suffer what I and others call a "misuse syndrome," similar to a repetitive stress syndrome, for which there are helpful therapies, including the Alexander Technique, which is a way of reducing tension in the body by becoming more aware of balance, posture, and coordination while performing everyday actions (I'll fully describe this method in chapter 10).

As I mentioned earlier, X-rays can provide clues for some patients who aren't finding relief otherwise. I recently performed a quick analysis of the X-ray reports from my last fifty patients aged thirty-five to sixty-five with "mechanical low back pain." The following three conditions, all of which are associated with age, are the most common observations reported by the radiologist (in clinical speak):

1. Degenerative changes with diminution in disc height. Translation: The vertebrae are closer together than they should be, suggesting that the discs have degenerated so that the space between the vertebral bodies is decreased.
2. Findings consistent with osteoarthritis. Osteoarthritis implies that there is new bone formation in a number of areas on the spine. These are sometimes called osteophytes, and are commonly referred to as bone spurs. They are nature's response to injury related to the aging process or mild trauma.
3. Facet hypertrophy. When the facet joints become hypertrophied, they are larger and more irregularly shaped than normal. This is also in response to progressive low levels of injury, which occur over time in the course of one's life.

The final three commonly reported conditions—*spondylolisthesis*, *compression fractures*, and *bony erosions*—are more serious diagnoses that require more immediate attention. I'll cover these in a later section. For now, let's get back to you and assume that you fall under one of the top three categories.

If your X-ray report mentions one or more of the first three items, they are the first clues to diagnosis. The interesting part here is that whether these findings are present or not, if you're still suffering from symptoms, it's probably time to have an MRI if you haven't already. Unlike X-rays, magnetic resonance imaging scans offer a richer picture, showing a better contrast between different tissues—and not just bone. They also don't entail radiation. MRI works by powerful magnets, and there are no known biological hazards associated with the MRI. It's important, however, to use these tests at the proper time and in the proper setting. As you're about to find out, diagnostic findings need to fit the symptoms. And they don't always.

Magnetic Resonance Imaging: Fair Warning

If you were to pluck any elderly men or woman off the street and put him or her into an MRI machine, you'd likely find abnormalities in those images taken. Why? Well, who doesn't have a few things wrong with them structurally by the time they're in their ripe old age? But if you were to ask those same people if they experience pain associated with those structural changes, chances are a good deal of them don't. Sure, they probably have a few aches and pains here and there, but overall they are healthy and as strong as can be expected. So, how do you distinguish between what the images tell you and what's really going on?

In a most provocative study published on this topic, a group of researchers led by Maureen C. Jensen published a report in the prestigious *New England Journal of Medicine* in July 1994 titled "Magnetic

Resonance Imaging of the Lumbar Spine in People without Back Pain." It marked the beginning of multiple studies that looked at people who have never suffered any back pain at all—and consistently more than 60 percent of these pain-free people show herniated discs in their low back. Jensen's study in particular found a high prevalence of abnormalities in the MRIs taken of fifty men and forty-eight women who ranged in age from twenty to eighty years old. None of them experienced symptoms, yet their MRIs told a different story:

- 52 percent had a single bulge. (A bulging disc occurs when the disc's inner material, called nucleus pulposus, moves beyond its normal parameters and pushes into the thick outer wall, called the annulus fibrosus, creating a bulge.)
- 27 percent had a protrusion. (A disc protrusion is when the disc bulge is still contained within the disc's outer wall, but has worsened and is pushing even farther into the spinal canal.)
- 1 percent had an extrusion. (A herniated disc means the disc's outer wall finally breaks open, allowing the inner nucleus pulposus to "leak out.")
- About 64 percent had intervertebral disc abnormality and 38 percent had an abnormality at more than one level.

Across the board for both men and women in Jensen's study, the prevalence of disc abnormalities increased with age; increased age was also significantly associated with the presence of more than one disc abnormality. Other studies since this one have confirmed similar findings: The precise relationship between degenerated discs and pain remains cloudy. For now, it appears that a new rupture or bulge causes pain, sometimes serious, in some people but not in others. If you have pain and a degenerated disc, the pain might come from the disc, or it might come from muscle tension, lack of exercise, or any of the other causes I've noted. Quite possibly it originates from a combination of factors.

That said, don't forget that MRI does have an important place in diagnosing back pain. As I've already detailed, the technology provides several advantages over other types of imaging. Unlike general X-rays, MRIs can provide a window to see high-resolution images of soft tissue, which helps a doctor to determine the severity of, say, a disc herniation. In addition, tumors, cysts, inflammation indicative of an infection, and abnormalities with the bones of the spinal canal may all be seen with MRI.

There are special types of MRI tests to consider as well. For example, gadolinium-enhanced MRIs can help evaluate patients with recurrent disc herniation after they've undergone surgery. When the chemical element gadolinium is given intravenously and MRI scanning is performed within approximately ten minutes of the injection, the gadolinium infiltrates the scar tissue but not disc tissue, thus making it easier to differentiate between the postoperative scar and another disc herniation. This special type of MRI may also be useful in seeing the difference between benign compression fractures and the serious malignant ones that point to cancer of the spine.

The overall lesson here is to appreciate MRI for its advantages over other scanning techniques, but also be aware that they don't always tell the whole story. Or they tell a story that may not reflect your particular pain. An MRI is just one clue to have in your repertoire to get to the bottom of your pain and address appropriate treatment protocols.

The Second Line of Action

Let's assume now that you've had multiple medical opinions, multiple X-rays, and MRI tests, none of which makes a specific diagnosis. You now come to me, and I cannot identify a specific therapy for your pain, either. What I do next is consider adding the following protocol:

A narcotic analgesic: I do this in order to offer patients a respite from the pain. Sometimes this respite resets the pain threshold and by doing so, other treatments may be more effective. There are also those patients in whom one class of narcotics is almost totally ineffective and need to be switched to another class of drugs. This may be a reflection of the number of receptor sites that particular individuals have in their brains or spinal cords. Even large doses of a drug will be ineffective if they have few receptors. But they may have large numbers of receptors to another analgesic and experience great pain relief.

- An antidepressant: Almost every patient with severe long-standing low back pain has some element of depression. Most patients will simply feel better when they are less depressed, even with the same degree of pain. In addition, many antidepressants also have a direct ability to suppress pain.
- An anticonvulsant: The thinking goes something like this: Injured nerves attempt to regenerate. But this attempt sometimes leads to the nerves' sending an abnormal signal to the brain, such as an abnormal signal from a brain cell that itself can cause a seizure. Using this simplified explanation, one can see why an anticonvulsant (i.e., a medicine that controls seizures) might play a role in pain control.

If I begin to use this class of medications, my patient is in the unfortunate position of transitioning from an initial episode of acute pain (or multiple self-limiting episodes of acute pain) to chronic low back pain. Most physicians, however, are unaware of this transition because it occurs slowly and insidiously, especially once narcotics have been introduced. But, in essence, by the time these drugs are entertained and prescribed, we are now dealing with a new disease.

One of the hallmarks of this new disease of chronic back pain is its sensation. Patients who transition to this type of back pain no longer complain necessarily of sharp, piercing pain. They now describe their back pain as dull and aching. In this instance, narcotics, especially oxycodone in combination with acetaminophen (sold as the brand name Percocet) or aspirin is particularly helpful. Because the pain that persists for long periods of time causes depression, an antidepressant may be added to the regimen, which can also help desensitize the perception of pain in the brain. And, as I've stated, an anticonvulsant may be particularly helpful with long-standing chronic pain as well.

My goal is to prevent this transition from ever happening. Because it's inevitable for millions of back pain sufferers, however, I've devoted two chapters to this transition, including a focus on what I call "failed back syndrome," whereby every possible treatment, which in many cases includes surgery, has been tried to no avail.

Now What?

At this point I've reviewed with you a wide variety of available therapeutic options. We've made the following four assumptions about your problem:

1. It's confined to your low back.
2. You've had several episodes, but the location and quality of the pain has not changed.
3. The frequency of the episodes may have increased, as has the length of the episodes.
4. You've had X-rays and probably an MRI as well, but the studies have been inconclusive.

The assumption we made initially is that the prime cause of your pain is a reflection of an inflammatory process due probably to the first two pain generators—muscle and soft tissue. I suspect that if you follow the recommendations I've made in this chapter, you'll find that they will provide relief and give your back the opportunity to heal.

Needless to say, if you reinjure yourself by either trauma or the trauma of misuse, the pain can return with a vengeance, and you'll need to restart your healing protocol. The fact that your pain comes in episodes is itself an important clue. If it's neither constant nor per-vading every aspect of your life, your pain has not become chronic. Once pain reaches the level qualifying as chronic, the challenges to finding relief become much greater, and the potential for finding suc-cess in treatment is unfortunately much lower.

But what if your pain isn't attributed to muscle and soft tissue? What if time and the treatment ideas lead nowhere? Then we have to move down the list of possible pain generators and see what else could be causing trouble.

ACTION PLAN

- Unless it's obvious upon initial exam that you have a serious med-ical condition causing your pain, be prepared to try a protocol of non-steroidal anti-inflammatories, muscle relaxants, and physi-cal therapy where appropriate. You may also be advised to lose weight (taking the weight off your back), to avoid activities that trigger your pain, and to ice your lower back when you experience a spasm. The goal is to give your back what it needs to heal on its own and prevent you from transitioning from the acute to a chronic phase.

- If your pain is not better, or perhaps has gotten worse, and more than six weeks have passed since the onset of your pain, then it's time to consider a second line of action. The upcoming chapters that detail the pain generators besides soft tissue and muscle will help you navigate other reasons for your pain—and other remedies. Use the information in the following chapters to understand these other conditions, consider your physical exam and imaging find-ings, and evaluate your treatment options with your doctor.

CHAPTER 5

Pain of Disc Disease and Foraminal Stenosis

A s you know by now, most low back pain symptoms are related to injuries of the muscles and soft tissues of the spine, including the ligamentous structures. And yet the term that most people associate with low back pain is *disc disease*. So, this is probably a good time to sort out some misconceptions and make important clarifications. The back pain generators we have discussed so far tend to cause pain confined to the low back and buttocks. The pain generators that I'll cover next are more likely to cause radicular pain—pain characterized as shooting, or radiating, down one or both legs.

If your pain doesn't originate in muscles or soft tissues, then your detective work becomes more complicated. We'll need to use the clinical information you enumerated in the checklist from Step 1, combine that with the findings of the MRI reports, and see if we can come up with a possible diagnosis. In essence, we, like all good detectives, are pursuing a smaller and smaller number of potential suspects. We'll do this by a process that involves provoking pain and seeking its palliation. The method is by no means a guarantee that you'll find your solution, and it's susceptible to the placebo effect, yet it can provide valuable information.

First, I'll discuss disc degeneration, and then move on to disc herniation. The former is a frequent cause of low back pain, either by the natural aging process or in the context of a traumatic event. The latter is the one associated with sciatica because the disc comes out of its normal anatomical position and puts pressure on the lumbar nerve roots, which can cause leg pain, numbness, sensory loss, and weakness. In the worst case, the compression affects the nerve roots that go to the bowel, bladder, and sex organs. These are listed in the "red flags" we discussed earlier. In the final part of this chapter, I'll cover a pain generator that frequently has everything to do with the discs: foraminal stenosis.

Disc Degeneration

Many of my patients have symptoms of both disc degeneration and sciatica, but what does this really mean? You'll recall from chapter 2 that the intervertebral discs are pads made up of fibrous cartilage that resists spinal compression and permits limited movements. They spread the load evenly on the vertebral bodies even when the spine is flexed or extended.

The disc itself is made up of two distinct components, the outer layer called the annulus fibrosus, and the substance within the annulus fibrosus called the nucleus pulposus. Each one of these components is ideally suited to its function. The nucleus pulposus is the water-rich, gelatinous center of the disc, which is under very high pressure when the human is upright. It has two main functions: to bear or carry the downward weight (i.e., axial load) of the human body and to

SINCE THE LATE twentieth century, research has suggested that chemical causes may play a role in the production of mechanical low back pain. Components of the nucleus pulposus—most notably the enzyme phospholipase A2 (PLA2)—have been identified in surgically removed herniated disc material. The PLA2 may act directly on neural tissue or may orchestrate a complex inflammatory response that manifests itself as low back pain and, when placed on a nerve, will cause sciatica. This suggests that there is a chemical mediator to the pain in addition to the mechanical compression.

act as a "pivot point" from which all movement of the lower trunk occurs. Its third function is to act as a ligament and bind the vertebrae together. The annulus fibrosus is much more fibrous (tougher) than the nucleus. It also has a much higher collagen content and lower water content compared to the nucleus. Its main job is to hold in place or contain the highly pressurized nucleus (the nucleus is pressurized for holding up the weight of the body), which is constantly trying to escape its central position.

In order for a disc to function properly, it must have high water content; this is especially true of the nucleus. A well-hydrated disc is both strong and pliable. The nucleus pulposus needs to be strong and well hydrated to do its job of supporting or carrying the lion's share of the downward weight of the body. With a healthy annulus strongly corralling a fully hydrated nucleus, the disc can easily support even the heaviest of bodies! As the disc dehydrates, it loses hydrostatic pressure, and thus the ability to support the axial load of the body diminishes. This causes a weight-bearing shift from the nucleus to the annulus. Now we have an overload on the annulus, which can lead to degenerative disc disease that results in the following conditions seen on an MRI:

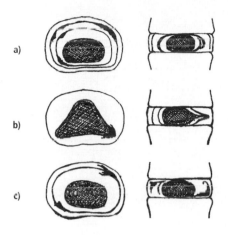

Three common types of annulus tears: (a) circumferential clefts, or delamination, (b) radial fissure, and (c) peripheral rim lesion. Disrupted tissue is shown in black, and nucleus pulposus is shaded.

1. Annular tears, of which there are three common types (see figure above). These become increasingly common after age ten, chiefly because the blood supply to the area decreases markedly after your early childhood.

2. Disc protrusions. If a rip or tear in the outer annulus ring is bad enough, it can allow the soft, nuclear portion (the nucleus pulposus) to bulge out. Some radiologists use the term *internal disc disruption,* or *severely degenerated* in severe cases, which are often seen in the elderly.

3. Endplate damage. Changes in the bone adjacent to the endplates—the interface between the cartilage and the bone—are called Modic changes, named after the radiologist who first described them. Some consider the endplates the spine's weakest link in compression; they can become rigid and unresponsive, and the underlying bone loses its ability to provide structural support. This endplate damage results in severe disc narrowing and the development of vertebral osteophytes, new bone formation in response to the damages.

But the question remains: How does this cause low back pain? The answer is that both the annulus and the endplates are innervated by small nerve fibers capable of sending a pain message. Discogenic pain typically increases with sitting, flexion, coughing, sneezing, and activities that increase pressure in the central portion of the disc.

If it's determined that you have degenerative disc disease, the general consensus is that the following options should be considered. As you can see, they go from least to most invasive, and can be done in sequence or in combination:

1. Physical therapy, which may include Williams flexion exercises, the McKenzie method, the Alexander Technique, the Feldenkrais Method, Pilates, and/or stabilization and strengthening protocols. This also includes nutritional management and core strengthening. (Although very few randomized studies support these methods in treating disc disease, those of us who treat this condition have seen patients benefit from one or more of these strategies.)

2. Non-steroidal anti-inflammatory drugs. This class of drugs is one that I use frequently because the response is seen quite quickly, usually in one or two weeks, and can be dramatic. Of course I check for allergies and side effects, and whether or not patients are on the medication for longer periods of time. I ask their internist to monitor the medication.

3. Cognitive behavioral therapy. This type of psychological therapy is most effective for patients whose pain has rendered them both physically and emotionally distraught. I devote more time to this devastating problem in Step 4.

4. Epidural steroids. Clinical trials on the benefits of epidural steroids don't match the impression of many practitioners. The risks of the procedure are small (consider the millions of women who safely receive epidural anesthesia for childbirth), but here again we have a case whereby some people respond and some

don't. Interestingly, a paper recently published in the journal *Spine* by a group of Stanford researchers led by Dr. S. Raymond Golish helps identify the people who respond well to epidural steroids based on the presence of certain molecules (fibronectin and aggrecan) in the spinal fluid. According to this latest research, people who have a complex of fibronectin and aggrecan in their spinal fluid are more likely to respond to epidural steroids. I find research like this very exciting, as it will predict those patients most likely to respond to treatment and save many others from the procedure.

5. Arthrodesis. Otherwise known as fusion, this is the treatment of last resort—when all else has failed. When the quality of the patient's life is poor *and* there are enough clinical and imaging studies to suggest that the patient will benefit from spinal fusion, this may be considered.

6. Artificial disc replacement. This strategy, which uses a totally artificial disc device, is relatively new and considered an alternative to spinal fusion. Because it can preserve motion, it can also minimize the risk that the adjacent disc levels will degenerate more quickly. There are a number of studies looking at this, and data is being published with results that don't seem to differ very much from those obtained with a standard fusion procedure. I suspect it will take a few more years before the final word is in.

Disc Herniation

One of the questions I am repeatedly asked is whether or not surgery is the optimal solution for treating a herniated disc. Lumbar discectomy, whereby the herniated portion of the disc—not the entire disc—is removed, is the most commonly performed surgical procedure for low back pain with pain radiating into a leg. But is it always necessary?

Surprisingly, more than a quarter century after the publication of the first randomized trial in this area, that question does not have a short or easy answer. Unfortunately, there have been very few randomized trials, and the evidence simply leaves much to be desired. Of the studies we can point to, however, a recent systematic review by a multidisciplinary group of authors found that the evidence favors surgery "slightly." Most of the evidence seems to indicate that early surgery in patients with sciatica provides better short-term relief of leg pain as compared to prolonged conservative care. One study in particular, published in the *New England Journal of Medicine* in 2007 and led by the Netherlands' Dr. Wilco Peul, demonstrated that early surgery in patients with six to twelve weeks of radicular pain leads to faster pain relief when compared with prolonged conservative treatment. The catch: There were no differences after one and two years between the patients who received early surgery and those who did not undergo surgery.

A second trial, which created much interest among my colleagues, was published by SPORT—the Spine Patient Outcomes Research Trial—and coauthored by a leader in the field, Dr. James N. Weinstein. That group found no significant difference in the outcome measurements between surgery and conservative care. But we need to be careful when drawing conclusions about Dr. Weinstein's study because it entailed lots of "crossover" patients. In other words, during the trial, some people who were part of one randomized group decided to switch to the other group; someone who was assigned to a nonsurgical group decided to opt for surgery instead, and vice versa. Such crossover activity could have skewed the results. So, it's no surprise that when the SPORT researchers further analyzed these patients in another study, they did indeed find better results in terms of pain and function among those who had surgery. Nonetheless, this observational study itself is still not easy to interpret.

One area that frequently gets addressed when it comes to surgery is cost. Is it more cost effective to intervene early with surgery than it is to recommend nonsurgical care? It turns out that surgery might offer an added bonus, according to Dr. Peul's study, which found that early surgery reduced work absenteeism.

Speaking of absenteeism, it's interesting to note as well that researchers have looked at one of the more high-risk types of jobs that is frequently met with back problems: professional football. According to a 2011 Northwestern Memorial Hospital study published online in the *American Journal of Sports Medicine*, it appears that undergoing a lumbar discectomy is *not* a career-ending event for National Football League linemen. A full 80 percent of the linemen treated with lumbar discectomy were able to return to play after undergoing the procedure. Of all football players, linemen are among the most susceptible to injuries involving the knees and spine; they are also uniquely vulnerable to disc degeneration because they spend a lot of time in a squatting stance, which puts tremendous pressure on their backs. The study's coauthor, Dr. Joseph Weistroffer, was quoted as saying how remarkable it is that "the numbers show they were able to get back to the extreme and sustained activity of playing football on an NFL level." If NFL linemen can recover quickly from back surgery and return to their high-impact game, then it's good news for regular folks who want to get back into the game of everyday life. It's also encouraging for people who are fearful of becoming active after disc surgery and continue to live like they did before. That said, the study didn't take into account a comparison of different treatment options and made no determination of long-term prognosis for athletes following their retirement. Nor did it address the very positive motivational attitudes of professional athletes and the strong financial benefits of returning to the playing field. In other words, future research will bear out these results and add more evidence to the debate.

When I help patients decide whether or not to operate for a herniated lumbar disc, it will, to some extent, depend on the severity of their symptoms and how long they have experienced the symptoms.

It's important to know that when a herniated disc causes pain, the disc can eventually heal spontaneously, by shrinking back to its usual size and sometimes by forming scar tissue that seals a leak or tear, removing the pressure on the nerves. Thus, even though we're dealing with an anatomical injury here—disc material exiting through a tear and pressing the nerve root against the bone, thus causing extreme back and leg pain—most of the time the body can heal itself within six to twelve weeks.

So, how does one decide to wait out the pain or request going under the knife? Rather than give you some hard-and-fast rules, which would be nearly impossible to do, let me instead offer a typical scenario and how I would think about the problem in an attempt to solve it.

Meet Mr. Smith. He owns a moving company. Three days ago he was lifting a piano with his team. He heard a pop in his back and immediately developed pain radiating down both legs. When he arrives in the ER, he complains that he is having difficulty controlling his bowels and bladder. The neurological exam confirms the finding and the MRI shows a large central disc herniation at L4-L5. This is considered a neurosurgical emergency and he is promptly operated on, with success. Had he entered the ER with the same history and even the same findings on the MRI, but lacked the problems with his bowels and bladder (what's called a neurological deficit), most physicians would have treated him conservatively with treatments that avoided surgery. And yet, if after six or more weeks his pain was still so severe that he couldn't function, then surgery once again would become an option. In a similar scenario, the pain would subside to a tolerable level following conservative treatment, but after six or more weeks, Mr. Smith would develop a persistent "foot drop," making it difficult to walk. (A foot drop is caused by weakness in the leg, leading the person to drag his feet around.) Here, too, the patient may be a candidate for surgery if the combination of time to heal and other modalities fails.

I hope that these scenarios give you a fuller picture of the complexity of the decision making involved. Disc herniation may be commonplace, but the exact method of treatment is not. Every potential solution must be determined on a case-by-case basis.

Foraminal Stenosis

The finding of foraminal stenosis is straightforward, but making the diagnosis is an entirely different issue. As you might remember from the earlier lesson on anatomy, the foramen is the "window" through which the nerves exit the spinal canal. Stenosis means simply that the window is smaller than it should be, and as a result, the nerves and accompanying blood vessels that supply nutrition to the exiting nerve are compressed as they leave the spinal canal.

The most frequent cause of foraminal narrowing is the accumulation of osteophytes, which again are small bony projections that develop with age, especially in response to multiple small traumatic events, which happen to almost all of us. This narrowing is similar to the narrowing we discussed in the development of spinal stenosis.

The other common factor that causes the foramen to narrow is the consequence of disc degeneration. If you look again at the illustration of the foramen on page 47, you'll notice that its height is the result of three structures: (1) the vertebra above, (2) the vertebra below, and (3) the disc between them. So, when the disc degenerates, the height of the disc decreases and the entire foraminal opening becomes smaller.

The challenge in making the diagnosis is that foraminal stenosis rarely presents itself as just foraminal stenosis. For instance, the accumulation of bone spurs is usually a sign of generalized osteoarthritis. And as you already know, this kind of arthritis is commonly caused by normal wear and tear as we age. Age-related disc degeneration can also be the culprit, or a combination of the two, each of which produces its own set of symptoms.

So, do you have foraminal stenosis? Following is a list of clinical signs that I would look for in a patient. See if these match your symptoms, as some are quite unusual:

- A positive Kemp sign: This means that if you bend toward the side where you have the pain radiating, the pain worsens. That is because the bending causes the foramen to be compromised even further. Patients with herniated discs also may experience this.
- Leg pain in the sitting position: This probably develops because the weight of the body itself causes further narrowing of the neural foramen.
- The need to limp on occasion, especially on the same side as the compressed nerve. This could be a result of the fact that the blood vessels, which accompany every nerve, are also being compressed. And when that happens while you're trying to walk, the blood supply to the nerve is compromised, causing pain.

The diagnosis of foraminal stenosis is based entirely on the combination of both clinical findings and radiological studies. Under the best of circumstances, the findings that I consider most important in making the diagnosis is an X-ray or CT scan that shows foramen compromise as well as the following:

- The compression is on the same side as the symptoms.
- The neurological findings and/or pain can be attributed to the nerve being compressed on the CT scan or on the X-ray. Remember that, despite overlap, each nerve has a relatively specific neurological function and distribution on the body's surface.

To reiterate: Foraminal stenosis is frequently a consequence to degenerative disc disease, which itself may not be limited to a single disc. Therefore, when the disc degenerates to the extent that it narrows the foramen, it will tend to do so on both sides and at multiple levels. Compounding this situation, a degenerative disc has abnormal motion. This motion causes the facets to react, and when the facets become abnormally enlarged, they will have further negative effects on the nerves.

It's no surprise that foraminal stenosis, like spinal stenosis, is an increasingly significant problem as more baby boomers develop symptoms with age. It's also no surprise that spine surgeons see foraminal stenosis in 10 percent of their cases for lumbar degenerative disc disease. This statistic is, in my opinion, also reflected in the large number of spinal fusion cases, many of which are said to address this problem. But many of these surgeries end up with patients who have failed back syndrome; they won't benefit from surgery and in fact may be worse off than before the surgery. Unfortunately, this group grows larger every year. Although I'll address this problem in detail later on, it's important for me to share the significance of failed back syndrome as it relates to foraminal stenosis. As much as I want to prevent you from going from being a patient with acute pain to one with chronic back pain, I don't want you to suffer from failed back syndrome, especially following unnecessary fusion surgery.

First, remember that foraminal stenosis is rarely seen in isolation, so it's often not diagnosed correctly. Second, the symptoms develop slowly over time; when most patients seek medical advice, their pain is quite disabling and in many instances they suffer from the inability to walk properly or fully engage in normal, daily activities. Third, we don't have any randomized control studies showing the effectiveness of certain treatments on foraminal stenosis. To some degree, I believe this is because most studies, such as those that examine the benefits of chiropractic, physical therapy, or distraction techniques, fail to single out patients with the specific diagnosis of foraminal stenosis. Again, patients with foraminal stenosis are normally lumped together with all patients who suffer from low back pain.

Because of these complications, one of the solutions that is routinely rationalized is surgery—namely, removal of the degenerative disc, and replacement with a structure that will restore the proper disc height and simultaneously reestablish a healthy foraminal size, which will take the pressure off those nerves. Such an "interbody device," as it's called, needs to fuse to the vertebra above and below, and most often is made of the patient's own bone. It also could be plastic or metal filled with bone. In order to accomplish this proper placement, a surgeon will place screws into the vertebra to stabilize the entire structure. These screws are connected by a rod to create a rigid structure. A good way to picture this in your mind is to imagine a carpenter gluing together two planks of wood using a C-clamp to stabilize the planks until the glue sets. In fact, the two vertebrae are fused.

This construction model makes sense. The building is collapsing on itself and the construction company is called to fix it, but it's not that simple! As with conservative treatments, we lack randomized control studies of lumbar fusion for foraminal stenosis to say conclusively that surgery provides a solution to this problem. Interestingly, a recent paper by an orthopedist at the Niigata Hospital in Japan suggested that the surgery I just described provided relief to patients with foraminal stenosis. This study reflected a very unique group of patients that underwent a procedure called the PLIF (posterior lumbar interbody fusion). The patients met very particular criteria in order to have the surgery; they had to experience not only all of the symptoms that I described for foraminal stenosis, but also significant neurological weakness as a result.

And therein lies one of the problems I see with patients who think surgery is their answer. It's unfortunate that the strict criteria used in the Japan study are not used by most surgeons performing this operation. This accounts for the rapidly growing number of spinal surgery procedures, particularly spinal fusion, many of which have poor outcomes. I'll explore this further in the last chapter of this step. Before we get to that, however, let's continue to explore the pain generators and turn to one of the most frequently diagnosed spinal conditions: lumbar spinal stenosis.

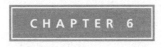

CHAPTER 6

Pain of Spinal Stenosis

T'S NO SURPRISE THAT spinal stenosis is diagnosed more often now than ever before, as our population grows older and lives with a much higher risk of suffering from this condition due to the realities of the normal aging process. The syndrome itself, however, has changed little since it was first described in 1954 by the Dutch surgeon Henk Verbiest.

The primary clinical hallmark is what your physician will call spinal claudication, and the easiest way to describe this symptom is as follows: You notice that as you walk, you develop low back pain—pain between the margins of the lower ribs and the inferior gluteal fold, the fold that separates your upper thighs and your lower buttocks. The pain frequently radiates into one or both legs and you have the sense that the farther you walk, the heavier and even wobblier your legs become. You might also notice that these symptoms improve if you stop and rest. After that, you'll notice that you're able to walk again with the development of the same symptoms, which again improve with rest. This cyclic pattern of pain with walking and relief with rest is often an indicator of spinal stenosis.

You may also notice that over the last several months or even years, the distance you are able to walk before you need to rest has gotten shorter. Many individuals with spinal stenosis also notice that the symptoms improve if they bend forward. In fact, a telltale sign is that when you go to the supermarket, you bend over the shopping cart, a phenomenon we'll discuss a bit more.

So, what is spinal stenosis and what are some of the ways it can be treated? In the simplest terms, spinal stenosis, you'll recall from earlier, is the narrowing of the spinal canal—the hole, or aperture, in the vertebrae through which the lumbar nerves pass. (To be clear: Spinal stenosis is the narrowing of the entire canal, whereas foraminal stenosis is the narrowing of just the foramen through which the nerve root exits the spinal canal.) Some folks are born with a small spinal canal, and this is referred to as congenital spinal stenosis, much in the way other body parts' size is inherited. But the patients I see usually have what's called degenerative or acquired spinal stenosis. They could have been born with a small canal, but regardless of their genetic predisposition, the canal has narrowed over time to the point where the nerves, and probably also the blood vessels to the nerves, are progressively compromised. In order to help my patients visualize this event, I ask them to think of a drain in their house that, over time, has become narrower due to the development of mineral deposits. The diameter of the drain gets smaller, limiting the flow of water. In a spine, this narrowing usually means that when the spinal canal is measured from front to back, which can be done on an MRI or CT scan, the canal measures approximately eleven millimeters or less.

The next most common cause of spinal stenosis is idiopathic, which is a fancy way of saying that we don't know why it developed in a particular patient. My own observation is that it does occur in fam-

> ## Is Your Back Pain Inherited?
>
> **ACCORDING TO A** new study from the University of Utah, symptomatic lumbar disc disease, a condition caused by degeneration or herniation of the discs of the lower spine, may be inherited. The study was recently published in the *Journal of Bone and Joint Surgery*. The researchers found that people with lumbar disc disease were more likely to have family members with the disease, and that the relative risk for lumbar disc disease was significantly elevated in both close and distant relatives. This strongly supports a genetic basis to symptomatic lumbar disc disease.

ilies and probably has an as-yet-unidentified genetic component. An extensive review of the other causes of spinal stenosis is something that your physician can go over with you once the diagnosis has been made, since the other causes are all exceedingly rare.

A condition known as spondylolisthesis also can cause spinal stenosis, but I'll save that discussion for the next chapter, as spondylolisthesis encompasses a unique set of circumstances and treatment. For now, let's turn to what causes the most common type of stenosis—degenerative stenosis—so that you can better understand this problem, from its concealed origins to its prominent and painful outcomes.

The Slow Cascade

Several factors, almost all of which are age related, act together to create this very common condition. What usually happens first is that, as with most of us, the lumbar disc degenerates over time and begins to protrude into the spinal canal, causing the first intrusion of the size of the canal. As the disc continues to degenerate and the disc height is further diminished, the protrusion extends farther and causes compression on the neural foramina (one of the pain generators that we've covered), leading to a condition you know is called foraminal stenosis. This puts a strain on the facet joints (again, another one of the pain generators). The facet joints respond to the increasing load by developing arthritic changes in response to the injury. As this chain of events marches onward, the joint and its capsule enlarge, causing a narrowing of the entire canal from the sides. This may result in the formation of a cyst, called a synovial cyst, which further compromises the canal and may also cause instability. All of these outcomes can cause the vertebrae to move independently of one another. As the height of the discs decreases, the ligamentum flavum (reviewed in chapter 2) begins to fold in on itself and stenosis is worsened even more.

A recent patient of mine demonstrates this complex array of issues well, and exemplifies one way of sorting this out. Mr. Gund is a fifty-seven-year-old teacher in excellent health. When I first saw him, he exhibited all the characteristics of spinal stenosis—namely, increasing pain with walking and relief with rest. What made his situation interesting is that he is an avid and longtime cyclist who can ride fifty miles with no significant pain, but he cannot walk fifty feet before he develops pain! I had met such patients before who obviously don't have vascular claudication since they can pedal without a problem and don't have traditional symptoms of spinal stenosis when cycling because they lean over the handlebars—flexing their spines and thus relieving their symptoms. Like the folks who lean over their shopping carts in the grocery stores, Gund leaned over the handlebars. In both instances, forward flexion opens the spinal canal and relieves pain.

Treating patients with spinal stenosis requires that the symptoms match the findings seen on the imaging studies. It's also important for your physician to rule out peripheral vascular disease. This is sometimes as simple as the physician's ability to palpate the pulses in your leg and foot; if there is a question, she will then do a Doppler study to confirm the diagnosis. A Doppler study is a simple test whereby a transducer is placed over the blood vessels to measure blood flow and pressure. Imagine sonar in a submarine and you get the idea. In Mr. Gund's case it was clear from the history that he didn't have peripheral vascular disease, but for many others in this age group, it's imperative that the diagnosis of peripheral vascular disease be considered.

The other condition that needs to be considered, particularly because it's also age related, is known as peripheral neuropathy, in which a nerve or group of nerves becomes damaged and can no longer transmit signals and messages effectively. Peripheral neuropathy can be caused by a number of things, including traumatic injuries, infections, metabolic problems such as diabetes, and exposure to toxins. Patients with peripheral neuropathy complain of numbness and tingling in their feet and legs, but the symptoms don't worsen with activity or improve with rest. If I suspect that a patient has peripheral neuropathy, I'll ask that electromyography (EMG) and nerve conduction studies (NC) be performed to confirm my impression. Electromyography is a technique for evaluating and recording the electrical activity produced by skeletal muscles, and nerve conduction studies give information about the nerves' ability to conduct an electrical impulse. This is important because my patients need to know that the symptoms of peripheral neuropathy will not improve with any treatment for their stenosis. But some causes of peripheral neuropathy are reversible, and many symptoms respond to medication, so making this diagnosis is important regardless.

The Options

My overall treatment plan for patients with spinal stenosis usually takes the following steps:

Modification of activities, if possible. Most people don't like hearing that they should change their level of activity. I don't recommend bed rest—it has no place in the treatment of this disease—but I do recommend that patients modify their activities so that they don't exacerbate their pain.

Integrative physical therapies that stress proper body mechanics. Many patients, for example, have benefited from the Alexander Technique or other similar practices (see chapter 10).

Drugs. Although some doctors will prescribe non-steroidal, steroidal, and narcotic analgesics; muscle relaxants; and antidepressants (or a combination thereof), I've had little success with these for patients with spinal stenosis. What's more, there are no studies that would support their effectiveness. So, I generally avoid offering medication to this group of patients in my practice.

Epidural steroids. The use of epidural steroid injections in the treatment of spinal stenosis is controversial. Although you won't find studies that show steroids work well, my clinical experience tells a different story. Admittedly, I haven't done a statistical analysis on my cases, but I have a large number of patients who have experienced long-term relief of their symptoms using this method, particularly after the first time they received an epidural steroid injection. Once the initial positive response wears off, though, it's less likely that additional injections will be helpful.

I should also add that as I write, new technologies are emerging that will help predict who can benefit most from steroidal injections. Recall the Stanford study I mentioned in the previous chapter that indicates we can know who will benefit based on proteins found in the spinal fluid. It's critical that the practitioner performing the injection has lots of experience in this procedure and that it be done with the help of fluoroscopy, an imaging technique commonly used to obtain real-time moving images of the body's internal structures through the use of a fluoroscope. In its simplest form, a fluoroscope consists of an X-ray source and a fluorescent screen, between which a patient is placed. Remember that epidural steroids are not curative— they are palliative.

Spinal spacers. There is a flood of interest in so-called interspinous spacers on the market as a treatment for spinal stenosis, and even suspected facet syndrome. You may have heard of some of these devices such as X-STOP, Coflex, Wallis, and DIAM. These devices are designed to fit between the spinous processes, which are located in the very back of the spinal column near the surface of the skin. In fact, by passing your hand down the center of your low back, you can feel several small prominences. These are the spinous processes.

Spacers aim to increase the diameter of the spinal canal and open the foramen, thereby "unloading" the disc. Since they can be implanted under local anesthesia, they have an intuitive appeal in people who seek a less invasive approach than standard surgery. There are several types of these devices, many of which are still in relatively early stages of development and testing, so data about indications for use, effectiveness, and potential risks and complications are often preliminary, and further testing is needed before conclusions may be drawn.

Others in my field share this opinion as well. In a recent blog post, Dr. Syed Kabir and colleagues, accompanied by a commentary by Dr. Adam Pearson on the Spine Blog for the journal *Spine*, suggests that patients and physicians withhold judgment on the clinical effectiveness of these devices because there is simply not enough evidence with which to make informed decisions about risks and benefits. The review makes it clear that, as with many new spine technologies, there is a lack of good clinical data regarding outcomes following placement of these devices. In one trial published in 2013 that compared X-STOP and decompression surgery (described next), doctors concluded that both treatments were effective procedures. But 26 percent of the X-STOP group required further surgery. This reinforces my suggestion that the X-STOP is a good alternative therapy with the understanding that a second, more invasive surgery may be needed later.

Surgery. When less invasive procedures fail, most physicians will recommend surgical decompression. This entails removing the osteoarthritic bone, hypertrophied or infolded ligamentum flavum, and protruding disc material. Removal of these elements opens the spinal canal. The challenge is to do so without removing too much bone, especially the facets. If this happens, the spine will be left unstable and might need to be fused. The results of three prospective trials, including one just published in 2013, indicate that surgical decompression is superior to conservative therapy, but here again the question that still needs to be answered is whether the results are long lasting. The data should be available soon, as the studies are currently ongoing.

There's no question that procedures such as the X-STOP and spinal decompression may be options when conservative therapy has failed. One additional note about devices such as the X-STOP is that if they fail to provide relief, they still leave the option of surgical decompression. So, at least theoretically, a patient can achieve many years of comfort and relief from symptoms with a combination of these procedures, and even longer if an initial trial of epidural steroids was effective as well.

Personal Values Come First

When Susan first came to see me, I was taken aback by her regal, patrician looks. An elegant woman in her late eighties, she had a younger woman's trim figure but the aching back more characteristic of her age. She had been referred to me by an orthopedist who, uncharacteristically, called me before her appointment to brief me on her case and make sure that I would "take good care of her." He had diagnosed her a few years earlier with spinal stenosis, and now all

conservative measures were no longer effective. Susan had been accustomed to traveling extensively to remote areas of the world, but
now found that impossible due to her back pain.

Susan lived up to the reputation that her referring doctor described
to me. Indeed, she had an independent-minded spirit and didn't want
to be seen as an old woman. It was quite clear on our first meeting that
she was having difficulty walking from the waiting room to the consultation room. She made every effort not to bend forward for relief
because, as she told me later, "that is what old folks do." Her orthopedist was indeed correct that she had severe spinal stenosis. I presented
her with options, and because of her age, I advised against surgery.

"Young man, I will decide what treatment is best for me," she
stated. Her surgery went superbly and I still receive her postcards
from exotic places. I learned my lesson again: Patients are still my best
teachers.

I also must add that I have had many patients, including young
ones, who have failed conservative therapy yet braved onward without
opting for surgery—even when I recommended surgery. These people
choose instead to continue modifying their activity levels and seeking
new conservative treatments. Some do eventually change their minds
if they don't find adequate relief. But many lead highly productive
lives without any invasive intervention and make peace with any re-
strictions that they have to bear. It is important to remember that not
all patients who undergo surgery do as well as others. As I've stated
throughout the book, surgery is never a guarantee. It might help you,
but it might not—and it could even leave you worse off than before.
Which is why the decision to go down that road should be carefully
thought out in partnership with your doctor.

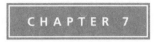

CHAPTER 7

Pain from Facet Joints

ETWEEN 5 AND 10 PERCENT of all people with low back pain
have facet pain, but if these percentages are stratified by age, the
cause of low back pain due to facets is nearly 45 percent in patients fifty to sixty years of age. As you know by now, a major clue
to this diagnosis is the fact that your pain is frequently unilateral—
one-sided. In fact, sometimes patients can literally put their finger on
the facet involved. It's frequently sports related or associated with a
specific activity. The pain can sometimes radiate down the leg, as it
did in my own case. But this can be confused with the radicular, sci-
atic-type pain. One distinguishing feature is that the pain rarely radiates below the knee.

Diagnosing a facet pain generator is made all the more difficult by
virtue of the fact that other pain generators in the lower back could be
at play simultaneously. Older people, for example, who have degen-

erative disc disease, foraminal stenosis, and/or arthritis in the spine are much harder to diagnose when it comes to their facets, because all these other conditions muddy the diagnosing waters.

Recall from the anatomy lesson you learned in Step 1 that the back is joined together by the intervertebral discs on one side, and by paired facet joints on the other. The facet joints can get inflamed as a result of injury or arthritis, and cause pain and stiffness. When the facet joints are affected in the neck or cervical spine, they typically cause pain in this area, as well as headaches and difficulty rotating the head. When facets in the lower back become inflamed, the result is low back pain.

Making a Diagnosis

As I noted earlier, one of the hallmarks of facet pain is its onset and how it feels. Three chief characteristics common in facet pain patients are the following: (1) the pain frequently comes on rather suddenly with an activity or trauma; (2) it's localized to one side; and (3) the pain does not radiate below the knee. That said, if the pain comes on more gradually, if you are fifty years or older, and if the pain follows the pattern of nerves down your leg, it may also be a clue that the facet is the culprit. In addition, many people experience more pain when they extend their spine.

Do X-rays help? Additional clues may come from routine X-rays, especially in older folks. X-rays can show large osteoarthritic joints that have degenerated. The same findings also can show up on a CT scan or MRI. I find the MRI particularly useful when it demonstrates fluid, which we call an effusion, a sign of inflammation in the facet. It is particularly useful if there are only one or two facets that demonstrate effusions or inflammatory changes and they are on the same side and location as your pain.

An interesting study done in 1976 by Mooney and Robertson is worth mentioning. These investigators used fluoroscopy to identify the facet joints in a group of asymptomatic volunteers. When Mooney and Robertson injected normal saline into these volunteers, it caused back and lower extremity pain. They then injected lidocaine into these "provoked" facet joints, and the pain was relieved. This experiment provided the basis for today's diagnostic testing to either confirm or rule out pain from a facet. We can selectively inject facet joints with a mixture of local anesthetic and possibly an anti-inflammatory steroid to see if there's immediate relief. And if there is, then a number of treatments may be considered, including more steroidal injections or radiofrequency denervation, a procedure that uses heat generated by radio waves to damage specific nerves and interfere with their ability to transmit pain signals.

The use of local-anesthetic blocks as a diagnostic tool, though widely used, has not been confirmed by randomized clinical trials. In fact, the treatments based on these diagnostic tests, which are widely used as well, have also not been confirmed by randomized clinical trials. Why is it important to point this out? Because this is yet another of the numerous examples of when the medical community uses a specific diagnostic test or type of treatment without solid clinical evidence backing it up from the research. In my own practice, I am faced with this dilemma every day, and the answers cannot be black-and-white. After all, I myself have walked off the table after a facet block and remain pain-free. If my physician had followed recommendations based on randomized clinical trials alone, I might still be suffering. What this further points out is that people are not studies, and every patient needs to be seen as a separate individual.

If your history and exam (and avatar) correlate strongly with the notion that you have a facet problem, your doctor will likely suggest that you undergo a facet injection for the purpose of confirming a diagnosis. What you need to consider before agreeing to this procedure is the person performing it. You'll want to find someone who does this on a regular basis so that he or she knows how to examine your spine for potentially painful facet joints at sites of maximal tenderness upon deep palpation. It is imperative that facet injections be done under fluoroscopy.

Let's assume, for argument's sake, that your block test is convincing, indicating that a facet is likely the culprit. Where do you go from here? Most patients who have a presumed positive diagnostic test for pain of facet origin are then considered candidates for steroid injections into the facet. This treatment was all the rage in the 1980s and 1990s (to wit, between 1994 and 2001, there was a 231 percent increase in facet injections, from 80 per 100,000 patients to 264 per 100,000 patients).

And then a randomized clinical trial published in the *New England Journal of Medicine* in 1991 threw a wrench into this option. The study cast a dark light on the practice, revealing that steroidal injections aren't as helpful as previously thought and could actually worsen the patient's prognosis. Despite my sounding this alarm, I've noticed a significant resurgence in the use of this treatment today, even though subsequent studies have at best shown moderate improvements in symptoms.

What's even more confusing is that critics of injections, while criticizing the technique, point out that no one has tested whether there might be a genuine benefit to patients who definitely have zygapophyseal pain. In other words, injections might help patients in whom one is sure of the diagnosis, but can be useless in those who may be suffering from a different pain trigger. Since, at the present time, the latter is not completely possible, it opens the door for many well-meaning and qualified physicians to proceed with the steroid injections and other modalities.

In my own practice, if I have a high suspicion that a patient has facet syndrome based on history and physical exam and there are further clues on the MRI, I'll make sure that:

- At least four to six weeks have passed since the onset of symptoms, so that Mother Nature gets the chance to do her magic. During this time, the patient begins with ibuprofen or progressive non-steroidal anti-inflammatory medication to control the pain that's generated from the secretions of substance P or prostaglandin. (I will usually prescribe relatively high doses.)

• The patient avoids bed rest but modifies activities.

• The patient considers physical therapy judiciously. There is no evidence that it is helpful in the acute phase, but for patients with progressive joint facets, I have found a number of different therapies helpful. Although there are no randomized clinical control trials to confirm my impression, the following treatments are safe and cost effective in the short term: spinal manipulation by chiropractors and osteopaths; in my practice I've found that this can be a very effective method of realigning the facets to their more normal anatomic position. The challenge is to keep them there after the manipulation. That is when certain physical therapies can help (see chapter 10).

What happens if you don't respond to these treatments, or your pain subsides for only a short time period—say, a week or two? If you've already had a steroidal injection, which is highly likely, then your doctor may want to inject you again. I, on the other hand, come from the opinion that second injections offer very little additional benefit. No procedure is without risk, and the administration of steroids needs to be done judiciously; for this reason, I usually don't recommend injections when other treatments fail.

If you were my patient, my next step would be to take a more invasive route and try ablating, or "burning," the tiny nerves that innervate the facet and its capsule. This is called radiofrequency denervation (sometimes referred to as a facet rhizotomy), because the heat used to burn the nerve comes from a specific frequency.

The results from this treatment vary significantly, depending on which studies you read. Some studies demonstrate a very high success rate, much higher than I would have predicted. In fact, a few studies

THE GOAL OF a facet rhizotomy, either a cervical facet rhizotomy or lumbar facet rhizotomy, is to provide pain relief by turning off the pain signals that the joints send to the brain. The pain relief experienced by most patients who have this procedure lasts months or even years, but results do vary. Patients who are candidates for the procedure typically have undergone several facet joint injections to verify the source and exact location of their pain. Using a local anesthetic and X-ray guidance, a physician will place a needle with an electrode at the tip alongside the small nerves to the facet joint. The electrode is then heated, with a technology called radiofrequency, to deaden these nerves that carry pain signals to the brain. Although rhizotomy is a minimally invasive surgery with very few complications or drawbacks, I'll admit that I was the exception: After getting the procedure myself, I experienced annoying numbness in an area over my thigh for six months. And in some people the relief is just temporary.

show that the success rate is greater than 50 percent after an initial radiofrequency neurotomy and upwards of 85 percent from repeat treatments.

As this book was being written, a group of Spanish physicians in Toledo published a paper titled "Identifying Patients with Chronic Low Back Pain Likely to Benefit from Lumbar Facet Radiofrequency Denervation: A Prospective Study." This timely report stresses my concern that injecting pain relievers into facet joints to diagnose true facet pain is prone to error, including a positive rate of up to 30 percent. The criteria these researchers used to identify patients with real facet pain entailed pain worsened by prolonged standing, prolonged sitting, twisting of the upper body, and bending forward. They also noted that relief among patients with facet pain came from rising, sitting, and walking.

The Spanish doctors also noted that among their group of patients that met these criteria, those who had a greater than 50 percent response to an anesthetic facet block responded well to facet rhizotomy. I'm hoping that these clinical clues may fit your particular situation so that if your MRI shows no other signs and you have a normal neurological exam, you may find relief from your facet pain with a facet rhizotomy. Your treatment plan won't end there, however. As these authors rightly emphasized in their paper, it's important to incorporate strength training into your recovery to boost your muscle strength, especially those related to your back.

CHAPTER 8

Pain from Bony Structures and Spondylolisthesis

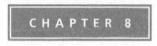

Back pain that originates in the bones of the spine is usually easier to diagnose, but the diagnosis associated with bony pathology is generally more serious. The hallmark signs of this pain generator include one or more of the following:

- Your pain came on suddenly or very quickly.
- A traumatic event or accident initiated the pain.
- You have a history of osteoporosis.
- You have a history of cancer.

The most common pain associated with back bones is an osteoporotic compression fracture, which means a person has suffered a crack or break in the spine due to the brittle-bone disease osteoporosis. Because of the link to osteoporosis, which itself is usually age related, this is seen mostly in females over the age of fifty. The pain is normally isolated to the low back, in and around the area of the fracture. Usually people who suffer compression fractures in other parts of their bodies seek medical attention right away because the pain is so intolerable. But for some reason, compression fractures of the lower back can be deceptive; in some people they can be equally as painful as a fracture elsewhere in the body, and in others, depending on the extent of the break, it can be just a mild to moderate pain that keeps them from seeking medical help right away.

A compression fracture is a clear indicator—it points to the fact that the bone of the vertebral body is weakened, in most cases by osteoporosis. In severe cases of osteoporosis the bones can literally collapse, so instead of their usual rectangular shape, the vertebrae look like a dented cardboard box. Often, they have a wedge shape, hence the term *wedge fracture.* Two serious problems that compression fractures typically cause: lots of pain, as you can imagine what a broken bone in your back must feel like; and the possibility that the collapsed and weakened bone is "retropulsed," or pushed backward into the spinal canal (bone fragments get physically pushed into the spinal cord).

About 700,000 cases of vertebral fractures triggered by osteoporosis are reported each year, the majority of which occur in the junction between the thoracic and lumbar spine or in the thoracic spine. Most patients do not give a specific history of trauma, but rather a relatively short history of moderate to severe pain. Clearly, the incidence of vertebral fractures increases with age. Other risk factors for such fractures include smoking, inactivity, and a history of falls and previous fractures. An additional risk factor that always attracts my attention is long-term steroid use. Steroid use implies that patients have needed to take the drug because of an underlying collagen vascular disease, such as arthritis, or a chronic obstructive pulmonary disease (COPD), such as chronic bronchitis and/or emphysema, each a chronic condition that in turn increases the risk for fractures.

In addition to osteoporosis triggering compression fractures, these breaks also can be caused by cancer cells, which we'll discuss later. Depending on the location of the fracture, either of these causes can stimulate spinal cord or nerve root compression and may result in a series of serious neurological problems, including paralysis of the lower extremities with loss of bowel and bladder function. If that happens, it constitutes a surgical emergency to remove the bone from the canal and to relieve the pressure on the spinal cord and nerve roots. This scenario is rarely seen with osteoporotic compression fractures, and is more common in cases in which there's a cancerous invasion of the vertebral bones or as a result of a traumatic event.

The Case of an Old and Broken Back

When I first saw Mrs. Edelstein, she had a two-month history of increasing pain in her lower back. At seventy-five, she had difficulty walking, and activities of daily living were becoming more challenging. Her pain didn't improve with ibuprofen or other over-the-counter medications. Her internist, who saw her before I did, noted that her neurological exam was normal, but since her last exam, a year previously, she was now one to two inches shorter and had a mild kyphosis, or curvature, in the area of her lower thoracic spine, which also had not been noticed the year before. When her physician palpated her spine, he noted that she had mild tenderness over the area of pain. Her doctor had ordered lumbar spine films, which revealed that the third lumbar vertebra had collapsed. It had the appearance of a crushed soda can, a finding consistent with a vertebral fracture.

It was also noted that she had generalized osteoporosis of the other vertebrae. Before she came to see me, I requested an MRI, but because she had a pacemaker, a CT scan was done instead. The scan confirmed that she had only one fracture and that the bones had not pushed into the spinal canal. A CT scan also ruled out the possibility that this was a tumor, either a primary tumor originating from the bone or a metastatic tumor that had originated elsewhere and ended up in the bone. With the diagnosis in hand, we were able to then consider the right treatment.

Treatments for Fractures Caused by Osteoporosis

Vertebral fractures are the most common manifestation of osteoporosis. Two-thirds of women with vertebral fractures have evidence of osteoporosis on the DEXA scan (dual-energy X-ray absorptiometry), which is a type of bone-density scan, and one-third of women have normal bone density on the same test. Some suggest that the postmenopausal women with low DEXA scores be treated for their osteoporosis in hopes that this will decrease the incidence of vertebral fracture. I will discuss this at the end of this chapter.

Fortunately for Mrs. Edelstein, the pain was tolerable. Many patients need hospitalization to manage their pain, yet data from randomized control studies is lacking to evaluate the efficacy of pain medication in this setting. In practice, however, NSAIDs and narcotic analgesics are commonly used. Some patients get minor relief with a rigid back brace. In my own experience, it's hard to tell whether the improvement of pain over time is due to the brace or the natural decrease in pain seen in most untreated patients.

Over the past ten years or so, the treatments of choice have been techniques known as vertebroplasty or kyphoplasty. They are generally referred to as vertebral augmentation procedures. The two procedures share the same underlying principle, namely the injection of cement into the vertebral bodies. This is done with large-bore needles called cannulae, which are placed into the vertebral bodies through tiny incisions in the skin. The cannulae are directed to their destination by intraoperative fluoroscopy. The procedure has been so popular that in 2005, 86 of every 100,000 fee-for-service Medicare beneficiaries underwent vertebroplasty.

With a percutaneous vertebroplasty, medical-grade cement is injected directly into the vertebral body. The cement is made opaque so that it can be observed under the fluoroscope. The aim is to reconstitute the normal vertebral architecture with the injection. Kyphoplasty, on the other hand, uses a balloon inserted through a cannula into the vertebral body. The balloon is filled with cement to re-expand the vertebrae and approximate its normal architecture. This latter procedure has the advantage of containing the cement within the balloon and minimizing the possibility that the cement will leak or spill into adjacent areas, which can no doubt cause serious complications if it ends up in the area of the nerves or the spinal cord.

By way of full disclosure, let me say that I don't perform either of these procedures. But I've seen a large number of patients achieve relief through both procedures, thanks to colleagues of mine who specialize in these techniques. If asked, I would say that these are highly successful procedures. Within days, patients can go from being admitted to the hospital in severe pain to walking the halls of the hospital—well enough to complain about the institutional food!

The Benefits of Vertebroplasty

It came as a surprise to me, and I suspect to a large number of other physicians, when the *New England Journal of Medicine* published two papers simultaneously in August 2009, each showcasing a randomized control study that found no difference between vertebroplasty and a sham ("fake") anesthetic injection for pain relief in patients with osteoporotic fractures. Both studies also reported that there was no difference in functional disability or quality of life among the patients. And of course these results were disseminated to the public when they were reported in every major newspaper and broadcast news outlet.

I highlight this controversy for good reason. You already know that one of my goals in writing this book is to present the most recent data based on randomized controlled studies, which are the gold standard in scientific circles. But, similar to other treatment options that I have discussed, this is yet another instance in which my decades-long clinical experience does not jibe with the published literature. As a physician and surgeon who has seen and treated thousands of patients over the years, I cannot just consider the academic wisdom. When I sit with a patient in pain, the advice and plan of action that I suggest are based on both evidence from the literature and my own experience. And sometimes they may entail going against the current thinking in academic circles. If I wholeheartedly believe that a patient will benefit from one of these procedures, then I will suggest it.

Without citing all the previous studies, let me say that there has been a subsequent randomized controlled trial comparing vertebroplasty with maximal medical treatment. This study followed patients for one to three years, showing significant improvement in the quality of life among people who received vertebroplasty. It also demonstrated that vertebroplasty can restore vertebral height and to some extent correct spinal deformity. So, here we have it: conflicting evidence in separate randomized controlled trials. My take-home lesson and suggestion to you as a reader who may be suffering from osteoporotic lumbar fractures are as follows: If your pain is severe and unresponsive to analgesics, consider undergoing one of these procedures. The complication rate is extremely low and it may profoundly improve your quality of life. If your pain is manageable, however, first follow a more conservative route, including analgesics, a back brace, and a modified physical therapy program.

It's also important to consider what steps you might take to increase the mineral content of your bones to avoid either an initial compression fracture or subsequent compression fractures. All current guidelines for managing osteoporosis recommend adequate intake of calcium (greater than 1,000 mg per day) and vitamin D (equal to or greater than 600 international units per day). That said, I'm sorry to report that no placebo-controlled randomized study has ever shown that there is a reduced risk of clinical vertebral fractures when you increase your calcium and/or vitamin D intake using these guidelines. Hopefully future research will bear this out.

Other options? Indeed, there are large randomized placebo-controlled double-blind studies in postmenopausal women showing the efficacy of several pharmacotherapies. These include drugs such as bisphosphonates, selective estrogen receptor modulators, parathyroid hormone, and then denosumab, strontium ranelate, and calcitonin. If you are the patient with compression fractures, then I strongly suggest you discuss with your physician which, if any, of these treatments may be best suited to you.

What Finding Bone Tumors Really Means

Pain originating from a tumor in the bone is rare, but when it occurs, it's more likely to be the result of a malignancy—cancer that originated in another part of the body and has spread, or metastasized, to the bones of the spine. Malignant tumors that originate within the bones of the spine are extremely unusual. In fact, I've never seen a case. I have, however, treated several cases of benign bone tumors. These so-called chondromas, as well as osteoid osteomas, typically present with pain, and the pain improves dramatically with the removal of these benign lesions.

Bone tumors tend to follow a pattern in their origin. In men, prostate cancer is the most common culprit, and in women, it's breast cancer. Other types of cancers can spread to the bones of the spine but are less likely to do so. These tumors weaken the bone and can cause the vertebral body to collapse. But, unlike the collapses caused by osteoporotic fractures, malignant tumors do not confine themselves to the vertebral bodies alone; they spread to the pedicles, laminae, and adjacent bony structures. In addition, they can completely erode the bone of the spine and extend into the spinal canal. And, depending on the location, the spread can cause compression of the spinal cord and nerves.

In order to treat these malignant tumors effectively, every effort is first made to identify the primary source (e.g., prostate, breast, and so on), as the treatment may very well depend on the origin or source of the tumor. Some cancers are best treated with chemotherapy, while others respond better to radiation therapy, or a combination of both. In instances when the primary location of the tumor is not readily identified, the spinal bone itself will be biopsied in hopes that the metastatic site will identify the primary site. In other instances, immediate surgical decompression may be warranted if the cancer is causing rapid compression of the spinal cord or nerve roots with an impending neurological problem or if the neurological deficit has already developed, which can be as serious as the inability to move.

People who land in my office with bony spinal tumors are always under the care of an oncologist, and surgery is the last resort. In such cases, early detection and treatment frequently increase both their longevity and quality of life. As for treating the many types of cancer, each year progress is made in extending the lives of patients.

Trauma

If you're reading this book, you're not likely to be among those who have suffered a broken bone in your back due to an accident or injury. Although trauma can cause back pain of bony origin, the nature of such injuries will have you in your doctor's office or ER in no time, and you will be quickly diagnosed, given the circumstances, and juxtaposed with your X-rays. For many years, I was neurosurgical director of spinal surgery at a major trauma center. The vast majority of our patients were involved in vehicular or motorcycle accidents. The others, such as the painter who fell off the roof, the hunter who fell asleep in his lair and fell out of the tree, or the convict who unsuccessfully jumped over the prison wall, all knew what caused their pain and, in some cases, neurological problems. It was trauma. Simple as that. Such diagnoses are typically a slam dunk compared to figuring out the complex subtleties of symptoms that reflect osteoporotic fractures or cancer.

Spondylolysis and Spondylolisthesis

Back pain of bony origin isn't just for those of us who are vulnerable to age-related disease and the ills of normal wear and tear over the years. Another type of stress fracture is the most common cause of low back pain in adolescent athletes, and it's visible on an X-ray. Technically, the condition is called spondylolysis (spon-dee-low-LYE-sis), and it entails a stress fracture in one of the bones. It usually affects the fifth lumbar vertebra in the lower back and, less commonly, the fourth lumbar vertebra.

If the stress fracture weakens the bone so much that it is unable to maintain its proper position, the vertebrae can start to shift out of place. This condition is called spondylolisthesis (spon-dee-low-lis-THEE-sis). If too much slippage occurs, the bones may begin to press

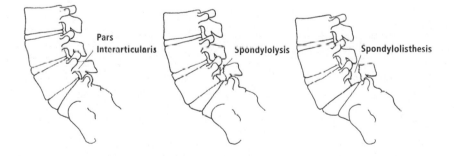

Left: The pars interarticularis is found in the posterior portion of the vertebra. Center: Spondylolysis occurs when there is a fracture or nonunion of the pars portion of the vertebra. Right: Spondylolisthesis occurs when the vertebra shifts forward due to instability from the pars defect.

on nerves and surgery may be necessary to correct the condition. As we'll see shortly, spondylolysis also shares features with two conditions we have already reviewed, spinal stenosis and foraminal stenosis. But I am including it in this chapter because it boils down to a simple stress fracture.

To think of spondylolisthesis in the simplest terms, consider the appearance of the spine from a side view. Although there are the normal curves, the vertebrae and the discs all line up pretty perfectly. Mother Nature, being the expert mason, has made a flawless column of bones (the vertebrae) and border (the discs). Now imagine that two of the vertebrae are not aligned. One has slipped in front of the other; this is spondylolisthesis—a word that's harder to spell and articulate than it is to diagnose!

Now consider the following: The vertebrae have an opening through which the nerves travel. If the bones line up normally, the diameter of this opening remains the same, but if the bones slip on each other, the diameter is compromised. The smaller diameter, in effect, is creating a narrower spinal canal. Now consider the neural foramen we discussed previously. Its size is dependent on the height of the vertebra above, the height of the disc, and the height of the vertebra below. If a vertebra slips, it causes a compromise in the size of the canal and may trigger the symptoms of foraminal stenosis. Because of this combination of events, 62 percent of patients with spondylolisthesis experience both low back pain and sciatica, 31 percent have low back pain, and 7 percent have sciatica.

The question then is, why did the bone slip and what treatment options are available? The three most common causes of spondylolisthesis are:

CAUSE #1: ISTHMIC SPONDYLOLISTHESIS

The center figure on the previous page demonstrates that there is a bony defect between the top portion of the posterior part of the vertebrae and the bottom portion. This defect is really a congenital nonunion, or nonfusion, of these bones. The defect in this bone—the pars bone—is called a spondylolysis and is present in 6 percent of the population. It's estimated that 75 percent of patients with spondylolysis will also demonstrate a spondylolisthesis. Because there is a nonfusion, the bone is held together by a fibrous band that, with time and/or with trauma, stretches, and the vertebra slips.

Gymnasts, weight lifters, and football linemen are particularly prone to the development of symptoms, probably because of overextension, overarching, and overuse. The pars bone fragment can become detached, compressing the exiting nerve root.

The good news is that most people with spondylolisthesis have no symptoms and don't even know that they have the condition. When symptoms do show up, they are usually in the form of general low back pain. Some patients complain of tightness and spasms in their hamstrings, which often cause a waddling gait—a short stride with the knees slightly bent. If the nerve is compressed, the usual radicular symptoms may also manifest themselves.

The degree of slippage is graded 1 to 4. Grade 1 is a slippage of up to 25 percent of one bone on the other; grade 2, up to 50 percent; grade 3, up to 75 percent; and grade 4, from 76 percent to a complete slip or 100 percent, when the bones can be seen independently or do not line up at all.

The greater the slip, the more likely you'll exhibit symptoms; conversely, with the lesser slip, you'll experience fewer symptoms and it's more likely you can be treated nonsurgically. We also know that it is probably only a small percentage of patients who progress from a lower- to higher-grade spondylolisthesis. To date, however, there are no ways to distinguish between the group that progresses and those who do not.

CAUSE #2: DEGENERATIVE SPONDYLOLISTHESIS

This is most commonly seen in people older than fifty. Patients do not have a defect/nonunion of the pars. The vertebrae in this group of patients slip because the facets that are largely responsible for maintaining spinal alignment become osteoarthritic and weakened. Most degenerative spondylolisthesis occurs at L4-L5 and at L3-L4.

As with so many potential back treatments, there are no randomized control studies for the conservative management of spondylolisthesis. Initial treatment for spondylolysis is always nonsurgical. I recommend that individuals with this diagnosis take a break from their activities until symptoms go away, as they often do. Anti-inflammatory medications, such as ibuprofen, may help reduce back pain.

Occasionally, a back brace and physical therapy may be recommended. In most cases, activities can be resumed gradually and there will be few complications or recurrences. Stretching and strengthening exercises for the back and abdominal muscles can help prevent future recurrences of pain. Periodic X-rays will show whether the vertebra is changing position.

Because few patients with slips of grade 1 and even grade 2 have a neurological deficit, the goal of treatment is pain control. Following is my protocol:

- In my own practice, if patients have an episode of acute low back pain, I treat them with the same regimen that I would treat almost any case of low back pain that doesn't have a specific cause: avoidance of the behavior or activity that causes the pain, especially in the groups I mentioned earlier who are at higher risk.
- Non-steroidal anti-inflammatories are frequently helpful.
- Judicial use of narcotic analgesics.
- I have also found that an exercise program or physical therapy program that stresses muscular strengthening and improved flexibility is helpful.

- A back brace for support, especially one contoured for the specific patient, also seems to ease the pain.
- In addition, I have had patients improve with chiropractic care, Pilates, the Alexander Technique, and the Feldenkrais Method. Other, conservative options may be helpful, but I have had no experience with them, and, again, there is no clinical trial basis on their behalf. Some of my patients have tried acupuncture with little or no success.

Surgery may be needed if slippage gradually worsens or if the pain does not respond to nonsurgical treatment and begins to interfere with activities of daily living. The patients with slips of grade 2 or greater can develop debilitating pain and a neurological deficit. Their cases are more challenging and frequently require corrective require corrective spinal surgery. The goal of such surgery is not too different from that of surgery for spinal stenosis: It's to decompress the spinal canal and reconstitute the disc height with an interbody device, which can open the foramen.

Two other goals of the surgery, especially in those cases when the pars segment is compressing the nerve root, are to remove that mobile piece of bone and to fuse the spine so that the slip does not progress any further. Of the few randomly controlled trials for the surgical treatment of degenerative spondylolisthesis, the most quoted is the study reported in the *New England Journal of Medicine* in 2007. When researchers compared patients who underwent surgery with those who did not, they reported that 75 percent of the surgery group rated themselves as having a major improvement two years later, whereas only 25 percent of the non-operated patients could claim such success.

The good news is that, in general, conservative therapy for mild cases of spondylolisthesis is successful 80 percent of the time. In more severe cases in which surgery is recommended, the success rate is equally strong, as upwards of 85 to 95 percent of patients have relief.

CAUSE #3: TRAUMA

A stress fracture of the pars is the most common cause of low back pain in adolescent athletes. Visible on an X-ray, it usually affects the fifth lumbar vertebra and, less commonly, the fourth lumbar vertebra. If the stress fracture weakens the bone so much that it is unable to maintain its proper position, the vertebra can start to shift out of place. Here, too, if slippage occurs, the bones may begin to press on nerves and surgery may be necessary to correct the condition.

Teenagers who complain of low back pain, especially those participating in strenuous sports, should have X-rays to determine if they have spondylolysis and/or spondylolisthesis. Interestingly, there is some evidence of a genetic component to spondylolisthesis. This evidence comes from examining fraternal and identical twins who have the defect, but as yet no specific marker has been identified.

WHEN IT COMES to back pain, if you can pin your pain on a faulty or otherwise dysfunctional anatomical structure, your battle is half won. And if you're diagnosed correctly and you receive prompt treatment (which can include a non-invasive, wait-and-see approach to let the body heal on its own), relief is usually right around the corner. But where we're going next is far from the world of "take *x* to remedy *y*." It's where people get lots of treatment but no relief. They are, as you're about to find out, victims of failed back syndrome.

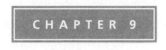

CHAPTER 9

Failed Back Syndrome

M Y WIFE REMINDS ME to avoid the word *hate*. "It's too harsh a word!" she says.

But I do hate the term *failed back syndrome*. So many patients who carry this diagnosis have the impression that they or their backs have failed, when in most cases, it's the medical system that has failed them! In general, failed back syndrome describes those unfortunate patients who had spinal surgery and have received no benefit, or, in some cases, they feel that their pain is worse after the operation. It's perhaps the worst place to be as a back pain sufferer. And it requires the attention of a full chapter on its own.

The primary aims of this book have been, first, to make sure you have enough information to advocate for the care you need and deserve. Essential to this process is that you're diagnosed properly with the appropriate diagnostic testing, and your treatment plan begins with the least invasive techniques, extending to the most invasive when necessary. In choosing an appropriate path, it helps to consider which therapies are based on randomized controlled trials, which ones are not, and how your value system plays into the choices you make. And second, to prevent you from becoming a chronic pain patient. Negotiating this dramatic change in your symptoms and treatment choices is not an easy task. Which brings me to this chapter, devoted to a formidable crossroads: You have had your surgery and you are no better, and perhaps even worse. What can you do now?

Unfortunately, many of you reading this book have probably been reading as fast as you can to learn the secrets to relief because you've fallen into this category. Many of you may also fall into both the failed back syndrome category and the chronic pain category. My goal in this chapter is to help you make some sense of your present predicament. Can you get to the bottom of your pain, and are there any options left for you to consider in hopes of finding relief or, at least, a management plan you can live with? Absolutely.

First Things First

Dealing with failed back syndrome may be a complicated issue, but if there's one simple fact for you to remember about this predicament, it's this: Failed back syndrome is not a single disorder, because it has more than one cause.

To start, I'm going to ask you to participate in an exercise in which I'll provide you with possible clues to your pain and you'll check those that pertain to you. This exercise assumes that most causes of failed back syndrome are a result of:

1. Improper diagnosis or improper reasons for choosing surgery.
2. Wrong or inadequate operation.
3. A complication from surgery.
4. Progression of the original pain or a new pain of new origin.

Ask yourself: How did your pain change as a result of your treatment(s)? Which of the following best describes you:

- The pain never went away. My procedures provided no relief whatsoever.
- I had some relief right away, but then the symptoms recurred. (This is sometimes referred to as an intermittent failure.)
- I had relief right away, but after one or more years the pain came roaring back. (This is called a late failure.)

Next, ask yourself whether or not the pain:

- Affects either one or both legs.
- Is essentially back pain.
- Is a combination of both.

Since the combination of low back pain and leg pain is so common, it is helpful to put a percentage on which pain comes from which area. In other words, how much of your pain, percentage-wise, is experienced in your leg as compared to your back? For example, is 40 percent of the pain in your legs and 60 percent in your back? This might help us determine your pain generator.

Needless to say, I cannot discuss every possible cause of failed back syndrome, so in this exercise I'll discuss those that are most common.

Wrong Diagnosis or Wrong Candidate for Surgery

Immediate failure caused by a misdiagnosis is actually quite rare. The goal in this small number of patients who fail to improve is to rule out potentially serious medical conditions that can imitate the pain. A missed tumor, for instance, is a particularly serious oversight. Some tumors—such as those of the bone of the spinal column, hip, pelvis, as well as soft tissue tumors and spinal cord tumors—can cause both leg and back pain. Even less common is pain originating from the kidneys or endometriosis, a condition that affects women when uterine cells grow outside the uterus and cause pain. Some of these diagnoses may elude the surgeon because they are not routinely seen as the pain generator. They are also hard to diagnose because they don't routinely show up on CT scans or MRIs designed to target the spine.

The most common cause of the immediate failure is poor patient selection. What I mean by this is that patients underwent surgery without a crystal-clear reason for doing so. Because this is such a common problem today, I insist that patients coming to see me because of persistent postoperative pain bring the imaging studies performed prior to their surgery. In many instances, this gives me more information than the postoperative study.

Quite frankly, it's disheartening to see how many patients fall into this category. The seriousness of this problem cannot be overemphasized. You don't want to enter what I call the medical vortex—when

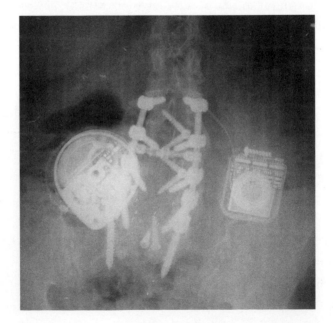

being an improper candidate for surgery leads to continued pain, which then ends in a series of further unnecessary surgeries.

The image on the previous page represents a real patient I saw recently. You don't want to end up like this. Mrs. Z had a work-related injury and developed low back pain. She failed all conservative therapies and was then referred to a surgeon. This particular surgeon typified too many surgeons out there—the ones I call Dr. Shuffle. These doctors perform one surgical procedure after another to address a house of falling cards. And it almost always turns out badly. In Mrs. Z's case, she first underwent a two-level lumbar fusion because her MRI showed some annular tears. She was absolutely no better after the surgery, so she underwent another fusion procedure using a different technique with rods and screws. The assumption was that in the first approach, what's called an anterior fusion, the construct was not solid enough. But because the original pretexts for surgery were incorrect, the second fusion also failed to provide any relief. The surgeon then went ahead to extend the fusion from L3 down to the sacrum. Still no better, Mrs. Z endured yet another fusion that was extended to the sacroiliac joints. Still seeing no improvement, she then had a dorsal column stimulator implanted, and went on to have a morphine pump implanted. She finally came to see me, still experiencing pain after all these invasive procedures!

It was clear to me that the woman was depressed and anxious. The chances of her getting better with the first of her many operations were small, because from the beginning she was never a good candidate for the surgery. The statistics on failed back syndrome reveal that almost one-half of the patients have psychological and psychiatric disorders that preclude a happy ending. This failure rate is even greater when patients with workers' comp injuries or active litigation are involved.

For those who deal with chronic pain, and are liable to suffer from depression as a result, it's unlikely that any further surgical intervention will help. In fact, in chapter 11 we're going to take a close look at what are called the "yellow flags"—signs and conditions that put you in a unique category of patients who will derive no benefit from further surgeries. Instead of scheduling more surgery, you need a multidisciplinary pain management team with a heavy emphasis on supportive strategies to boost your psychological needs and regulate your medication.

Based on my experience, other possible reasons for postoperative failure include:

- Patients whose pain doesn't have a clear pain generator on any imaging study yet who clearly have neurological issues, such as weakness, numbness, or sensory loss, may have an underlying problem *unrelated* to spinal nerve root compression. Included in this category are exposures to various environmental or occupational toxins as well as common metabolic diseases such as diabetes or infectious sources such as Lyme disease, herpes, and others.
- Patients who demonstrate muscle weakness, but don't experience pain, need to see a neurologist to rule out motor neuron disease, commonly referred to as a motor neuron disease/amyotrophic lateral sclerosis (ALS), or Lou Gehrig's disease.
- Patients who have symptoms of spinal stenosis need to have a vascular workup to rule out vascular claudication. This workup should include electromyography to test the electrical activity of the muscles and rule out a peripheral neuropathy (see pages 108 and 109 for more on these conditions).

Wrong or Inadequate Surgery

An improper or inadequate operation encompasses a variety of different issues. Wrong operation implies that the indications of the surgery were incorrect. This can happen to the best of surgeons. What the responsible surgeon will do if your symptoms do not improve is investigate further, discuss your situation with his or her colleagues, and share their findings and thought process with you, the patient. It's important that you are involved in the diagnosis.

Wrong operation can also mean that there was an operative oversight or error. It used to be that the most common cause of malpractice for spinal surgery was operating on the wrong area, such as the wrong vertebra. Fortunately, this error is much less common today, thanks to mandatory standards in place to prevent such unfortunate circumstances.

In my experience, the most common cause of pain that does not resolve in the immediate postoperative period is due to inadequate decompression. In the case of a herniated disc, for example, a portion of the disc compressing the root has not been adequately removed. Another reason could be the fact that two disc herniations are present. This occurs in 15 percent of cases and the surgeon has made the incorrect assumption as to which one of the herniations is causing the pain.

In all of these scenarios, the diagnosis can usually be made with a postoperative MRI or CT scan. When failure occurs, it should be worked up immediately. The goal, once again, is to avoid additional surgeries and sending you deeper into the vortex of failed medical and surgical management.

Surgical Complications

Complications from surgery are very unusual and occur in less than 5 percent of cases. But I also believe that this percentage has been increasing due to the growing volume of both complex and minimally invasive spinal surgeries. With each one of these procedures, there is a learning curve inherent for a surgeon to master new technology. Clearly, a new driver is more likely to get into an accident than an experienced driver.

First, you'll want to make sure that your surgeon has enough experience with your type of surgery so that he or she is already way beyond that learning curve. Second, if your surgery entails implants or interbody devices or rods and screws, and so forth, these can also lead to what are called man-made pain generators, a phenomenon I will further discuss shortly. I also mentioned the fact that when two spinal segments are fused, and those two segments fail to fuse properly, it places additional stress on the adjacent segments, be they discs or facets. These other anatomical segments are now more likely to cause pain, a phenomenon called adjacent segment disease.

Patients who wake up from surgery that does not involve the addition of "hardware" to your back (such as screws and rods) and who have the same or worse pain usually continue to suffer for the following possible two reasons: (1) There was excessive traction on the nerve root during the surgery and the nerve swelled, causing pain. One clue to this event is that patients frequently develop a deep burning pain that was not present prior to the surgery, but is in the same place as their preoperative pain. And (2) the nerve was actually damaged during the surgery and/or the dura (the protective layer surrounding your spinal cord to keep in spinal fluid) was violated, causing spinal fluid to leak out. If the dura is compromised, it will require speedy repair during surgery.

If this describes your situation, you need to discuss this with your surgeon. Postoperative studies are usually not helpful in these situations, except when they show a collection of spinal fluid or possibly even the postoperative collection of blood. Either of these can cause compression of the nerve root or other structures of your spinal cord— namely, the thecal sac (the dural membrane that protects your nerve roots) and cauda equina, which mimics the symptoms you originally had. The cauda equina ("horse's tail") is a bundle of spinal nerves and nerve roots that resemble a horse's tail.

Patients who wake up with increased pain after surgery that involved the implantation of hardware (these are known as instrumented cases) need immediate imaging to assure the surgeon that the rods, screws, and interbody devices were placed properly and are not pressing against the nerve roots or thecal sac.

If you have no relief and increasing pain during this time period, other things your doctor needs to consider are:

- Infections, which can occur as early as ten days postoperatively.
- Loose or misplaced hardware.
- A fluid cyst.
- Recurrent disc herniations.

Pain That Returns Later

Not again! The most common cause of recurrent radicular pain— radiating leg pain caused by a herniated disc—after undergoing a microdiscectomy is another disc herniation. In some cases, this surgery involves removing the portion of the disc that is applying pressure to the nerves. It requires that the surgeon make an incision in the annulus fibrosus, the outer layer of the disc, to access the nucleus pulposus, the herniated tissue. In other cases, a tear in the annulus allows surgeons easy access to the herniated tissue. However, the disc can reherniate through the annular opening as it heals, resulting in the recurrence of pain and requiring additional surgery.

The incidence of recurrent disc herniation is about 5 percent. A smaller number of patients will develop epidural fibrosis, or what is commonly called scar tissue that compresses the nerve root. In my opinion, this is an overdiagnosed culprit. I routinely see some degree of fibrosis in almost all postoperative cases, but rarely am I convinced that it's causing pressure on the nerve. This is an important point, because the presence of fibrosis on the postoperative MRI gives justification to a wide variety of surgical and nonsurgical interventions, which are invariably unnecessary. If you have this diagnosis, my suggestion is that you ask your surgeon whether the fibrosis is actually causing nerve root compression, because fibrosis in and of itself, in my opinion, is not a pain generator.

When the pain recurs later, these can be easier to diagnose. If the symptoms include radiating pain down the leg, a recurrent disc is still high on the list of possibilities. But in instrumented/fusion patients, the list is longer and includes the following possibilities:

- Pseudoarthrosis, a fancy word that means the fusion never healed or it fused incompletely.
- The fusion fractured. Most patients in this situation have a history of postoperative trauma.
- Loosening of the hardware. This is particularly common in those cases where the fusion never healed or the fusion fractured, or in patients with osteopenia, and has a high incidence among smokers.
- Adjacent segment disease or facet pain now becoming the pain generator and the adjacent segment develops instability.

As you can imagine, all of these circumstances can be treated, but each will require its own clear diagnosis and course of action to remedy.

ACTION PLAN: SPECIAL NOTE

The prevalence of failed back syndrome today compels me to end Step 3 with two other items to underscore here. One, we live in a world where the majority of the population is older. I've seen lots of patients who suffer from failed back syndrome. For example, I've seen patients who have redeveloped the signs and symptoms of spinal stenosis following their initial treatments. A repeat examination reveals that they have a return of the stenosis usually near the original level (at an adjacent level). I cannot stress enough here, as I've been doing all along in this book, the importance of getting a proper diagnosis.

You don't want to end up with multiple failed surgeries and becoming the proverbial back cripple. Remember, the same principles of diagnosis and treatment apply to the postoperative patient as they do to the preoperative patient.

Last, be an educated patient. Find your set of circumstances and scenarios in the descriptions I've outlined and discuss the possible diagnoses with your doctor or another doctor until the diagnosis and treatment plan make sense. After all, this isn't astrophysics. The anatomy and biomechanics of the spine are really quite straightforward. If the doctor cannot explain to you what is going on, then I would question if indeed there really is a clear answer. And you deserve explicit answers.

Step 4

Embrace Various Pathways to Healing:
A Physical and Emotional Journey

BY THIS POINT IN THE BOOK, YOU'VE ALREADY BEEN INTRODUCED to a wide array of diagnostic tools and treatment options. You've gained an enormous amount of knowledge about the anatomy and biology of pain, and you may have nailed down your unique problem. In this next step, we're going to review all of the therapies that are likely available to you. This will include a discussion of both traditional and complementary strategies, with the emphasis on the likelihood that your cure will entail a combination of techniques—with or without surgery. In a chapter aptly titled "The Trail from Acute to Chronic," we'll see how easy it is to be transformed from the patient with what appears to be a single treatable problem to one who suffers from chronic pain and related conditions that severely cut one's quality of life in half, if not more. This is what I would like to prevent. I'll share a cautionary tale, and offer strategies to ensure this doesn't happen to you.

I'm also going to spend time in this important step equipping you with the facts of a reality we've barely considered yet, one that dovetails with the conversation about going from acute to chronic: what to do when the pain is rooted more in the psychological mind than in the physical body. The intangible perception of pain is as much a player in the pain equation as is your tangible anatomy and biology. I'm going to present an eye-opening look at the latest breakthrough in science about understanding pain and how the mind can sabotage even the most well-intentioned person who wants relief. You'll be asked to consider questions about your pain that you likely never thought to ask, such as: Does your pain serve you in some positive way? As before, it helps to read all of the chapters in this step and take each set of questions or exercises seriously. The information you learn in this step will reinforce all previous steps and get you on the right pathway to healing.

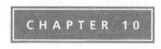

CHAPTER 10

Physical and Integrative Therapies

OW TIMES HAVE CHANGED! When I went to medical school
some forty years ago, the words *alternative, complementary, holistic,* and *integrative medicine* were unknown. There was no
such thing as "mind-body" medicine. In fact, practitioners of Western
medicine looked with disdain, even hostility, at those practitioners of
complementary modalities. Most of this attitude stemmed from igno-
rance. To think that Eastern practices, including acupuncture and
herbal medicine, which have been practiced for two thousand years,
had nothing to offer our patients was hubris. While some like to argue
that "alternative" is code for quackery, dubious and implausible, I beg
to differ.

My own eyes were opened when, as a resident, I watched a surgeon perform a thoracotomy—a surgical incision into the chest
wall—on a patient who was awake and given acupuncture as the sole

anesthetic agent. Later, at a lecture I attended, a Chinese physician pointed out that so many of the medications that doctors use daily are derived from plants and herbs. In fact, almost all of the major pharmaceutical companies spend large sums on research and development of new pharmaceuticals from plant life, sending researchers into the farthest corners of the planet, in places such as the Amazon and Africa. In these regions, many of the native peoples have been benefiting from these natural secrets for centuries, if not millennia. It is no wonder that many of these integrative treatments have become a part of the usual armamentarium of modalities to treat low back pain.

Developers of new drugs aren't the only ones searching for "alternative" ingredients for their formulas. Complementary, or integrative, medicine has been a growing aspect of medicinal healing as the general public becomes more interested in different aspects of natural living. When I was in medical school, purely conventional treatments were discussed. Thankfully, in my lifetime, I've watched the medical community embrace a combination of both conventional and integrative treatments, as now a significant number of medical schools offer elective courses in integrative medicine. In fact, according to a new study from the *Archives of Internal Medicine* (now called *JAMA Internal Medicine*) published in 2011, more and more American doctors are recommending mind-body therapies to their patients. Looking at data from a survey of more than 23,000 US households, the authors found that one in thirty Americans using mind-body therapies had been referred by a medical provider. And when it comes to back pain, an increasing number of both doctors and their patients are becoming receptive to the option of complementary treatment.

Integrative therapies are as diverse in their foundations as they are in their methodologies. Practices may incorporate or base themselves on traditional medicine, folk knowledge, spiritual beliefs, or newly conceived approaches to healing. In response to the growing demand for knowledge on integrative therapies, the National Center for Complementary and Alternative Medicine (NCCAM), an institute of the

National Institutes of Health (NIH), was created in 1992 because consumers of complementary and alternative medicine and health care practitioners alike wanted to know whether available integrative medical options were safe and effective. It studies modalities such as naturopathy, chiropractic, herbs, traditional Chinese medicine, Ayurveda, meditation, yoga, tai chi, guided imagery, biofeedback, hypnosis, homeopathy, deep breathing exercises, acupuncture, and nutrition-based therapies, in addition to a range of other practices.

It would be impossible to cover every type of integrative therapy available down to every minute detail. Such an endeavor would take up volumes of books. This chapter intends to provide you with a shorthand gallery of options that you will undoubtedly encounter on your road to recovery. I've already mentioned some of these therapies, and you'll find referrals to them again in future chapters. I thought it best, however, to organize all of the treatment ideas here so you can also use this chapter as a reference guide. First, I'm going to start with the more traditional options under the realm of physiatry, which refers to physical medicine and rehabilitation. Then I'll dive into the integrative side and review with you those treatments that I still recommend in conjunction with physical therapy. I'll also share what is known about their effectiveness, and in which types of patients they are known to work best.

One caveat to mention: Here again, we encounter the problem of nomenclature, since most studies do not distinguish the source of the low back pain—that is, they make no effort to identify the pain generator, and patients are lumped into the general rubric of "low back pain." Most studies will eliminate those patients with radicular symptoms and some will distinguish between patients whose low back pain is acute and those with pain of longer or chronic duration. What's more, some of the therapies I will cover, such as chiropractic care, are relatively recent treatments. Others are thousands of years old.

It's quite possible that the general acceptance of integrative techniques—coupled with sound studies backing their use—will not only change people's perspective on these options but will also negate the term *alternative* altogether. Many of these strategies will simply become part of the overall conversation in traditional medical circles. In other words, they will become part of mainstream medicine. As Richard Dawkins, an evolutionary biologist, describes it, "There is no alternative medicine. There is only medicine that works and medicine that doesn't work."

Physiatry (Physical Medicine) and Physical Therapy

LUMBAR STABILIZATION EXERCISES

Contrary to what the term implies, lumbar stabilization is an active form of exercise used in physical therapy. It is designed to strengthen muscles to support the spine and help prevent lower back pain. Through a regimen of movements, and with the initial help of an experienced physical therapist, you are trained to find and maintain your neutral spine position. The back muscles are then exercised to teach the spine how to maintain its position.

This exercise technique relies on something called proprioception, which is the awareness of where your joints are positioned. Performed on an ongoing basis, lumbar stabilization exercises can help keep the back strong and well positioned. It's a multicomponent program and involves education/training, strength, flexibility, and endurance. It's generally used during every phase of a back pain episode and may be prescribed after a thorough evaluation of your specific condition. Note that there is no one-size-fits-all in lumbar stabilization. Your physical therapist will help you design a program suitable to your needs and limitations. The goal is to teach you proper technique so that you can perform the exercises on your own. Lumbar stabilization has been known to help a wide variety of back pain sufferers, from those with muscle strains and torn ligaments to people with other pain generators. The exercises can help you gain control over the movements of, and forces acting on, your spine during daily activities, as well as reduce the chance of more back injury due to repetitive motions or sudden movements or stresses.

So, what is a neutral spine? While not necessarily pain-free, a neutral spine is defined as the least painful yet biomechanically sound posture for the lower back. This means it decreases tension on the spine-related ligaments and joints; it allows the various forces acting on the discs and vertebrae to be distributed in a more balanced manner; it keeps your posture near your "center," enabling you to react more quickly (either forward or backward) when necessary; and it provides the greatest functional stability with axial loading. In physics, axial loading refers to a load falling along the length of a lever, which in this case is the spine. Lumbar stabilization exercises ultimately help your back to carry the weight of the body, that is, the "axial load" of the body.

A PHYSICAL THERAPIST can show you how to align your spine and provide you with exercises to both strengthen your core and loosen up stiff neck, back, arm, and leg muscles (tight hamstrings can contribute to back pain). Move Forward (www.move forwardpt.com), a website of the American Physical Therapy Association, offers a simple tool that lets you search for physical therapists by ZIP code and specialty. Most insurers cover physical therapy, although some may insist that you get a referral from a physician before they will authorize a visit. If you decide to go out of network or to bypass your insurer, you'll pay $150 to $250 for an initial assessment. Follow-up visits will be $50 or so less. Although many experts say you can address basic posture issues in just one to three sessions, it's more realistic that you'll need multiple sessions over the course of several weeks to see an improvement.

Once learned, the lumbar stabilization exercise program is designed to train the muscles to maintain this neutral spine position subconsciously, quickly, and automatically. It will go a long way to help you to maintain excellent posture, which, as we'll see in Step 5, is key to back health.

WILLIAMS FLEXION EXERCISES

Paul Williams first published his exercise program in 1937 for patients with chronic low back pain upon noticing that the majority of people who experienced low back pain had degenerative changes as a consequence of degenerative disc disease. He developed his exercise protocol especially for people whose X-ray films showed decreased disc space between lumbar spine segments (L1-S1), and whose symptoms were chronic but low-grade. These exercises were performed with the goal of reducing pain and providing lower trunk stability by actively developing the abdominals, buttocks, and hamstring muscles, as well as passively stretching the hip flexors and lower back (sacrospinalis) muscles.

For many years, Williams flexion exercises have been a cornerstone in the management of lower back pain and treating a wide variety of back problems, regardless of diagnosis or chief complaint. In many cases they are used when the exact cause of the back pain is not known or, at best, is poorly defined. Many physical therapists will teach these exercises with their own modifications. I'll cover more specifics of these exercises in Step 5.

MCKENZIE EXTENSION EXERCISES

These back exercises are named after the late Robin McKenzie, a physical therapist in New Zealand who found that extending the spine through exercise could reduce pain generated from a compromised disc space. Theoretically, extension exercises may also help reduce the herniation of the disc itself and reduce pressure on a nerve root. There is a wide range of McKenzie exercises, some of which are done standing up, while others are performed lying down. All of these upper and lower back exercises use core muscle contraction and, usually, arm motions to stabilize the trunk and extend the spine.

For patients who are suffering from leg pain due to a disc herniation (a radiculopathy), extending the spine with McKenzie back exercises may also help reduce the leg pain by moving the pain from the leg to the back. The reasoning goes that back pain is usually more tolerable than leg pain, and if you can centralize your pain, you may be able to continue with nonsurgical treatment (such as exercise) and avoid a surgical discectomy.

When the pain is acute, the exercises should be done frequently (every one to two hours). To be effective, patients should try to avoid flexing the spine (bending forward) while exercising, as this undercuts the strengthening motion.

McKenzie exercises may also be helpful for those individuals who have back pain due to degenerative disc disease. Although sitting or flexing forward can accentuate low back pain for patients with degenerative disc disease, extending the spine can serve to relieve the pressure on the disc. Note that the opposite is true in elderly patients who have facet osteoarthritis and/or lumbar stenosis. Extending the spine jams the facet joints on the back and increases pressure across the joints, so these patients will typically feel better sitting, and have more pain with extension. As with the Williams exercises, I'll offer more specifics of performing these exercises in Step 5.

MYOFASCIAL RELEASE

Myofascial pain syndrome (MPS) is a fancy way to describe muscle pain. It refers to pain and inflammation in the body's soft tissues. Hence, myofascial release is a form of soft tissue massage therapy that involves stretching and manipulating the connective tissue, or fascia, of the body. *Fascia* is the technical term for the thin, fibrous tissue enclosing muscles and other organs. Fasciae are unique in that they cover and connect all of the body's muscles and bones. Because of this relationship with the body, trauma, inflammation, scarring, and repetitive stress can cause tightening of the fasciae—resulting in abnormal pressure on other parts of the body, such as the nerves, vessels, and organs. Myofascial release works to alleviate these tensions and knots and soften the tissue, often by the application of pressure from the therapist's hands to the fasciae. This therapy is commonly used to treat recurring sports injuries, headaches, neck and back pain, and recurring emotional and physical pain, as well as to increase flexibility and mobility.

There are two main types of myofascial release: direct and indirect. In direct myofascial release, the practitioner uses his or her knuckles and elbows and works directly on the affected area with high force to stretch the fascia. As you may rightly guess, this falls under the category of deep tissue massage. The goal is to change the structure of the fascia through stretching, pulling, and releasing adhesions, which are fibrous bands that form between tissues and organs and can be thought of as internal scar tissue. Indirect myofascial release is the lighter, gentler version with much less pressure applied to encourage the fascia to unwind itself without having to physically force it.

TRIGGER POINT INJECTIONS (TPI)

Trigger points are common sites for chronic and acute pain, even pain not associated with the back per se. Trigger points are basically knots of muscle that form when muscles do not relax. They can irritate the nerves around those muscles and cause pain that can be felt not only where they are touched and depressed, but in other parts of the body ("referred pain"). The term *trigger point* was first used in 1940 by Arthur Steindler, an orthopedic surgeon, yet the person most famous for defining trigger points through systematic studies is Janet G. Travell. It's no coincidence that Dr. Travell was the White House physician during the Kennedy administration and again during the Johnson years, two presidents who suffered from low back pain. Dr. Travell's extensive body of research has given us a clearer understanding about where trigger points are located and how they produce patterns of pain.

Trigger points help define myofascial pain syndrome, and they are classified as active or latent. An active trigger point causes pain at rest; it's tender to the touch with a referred pain felt elsewhere and that seems like it's spreading. This referred pain is an important characteristic of a trigger point. It differentiates a trigger point from a tender point, which is associated with pain at only the site of touch.

A latent trigger point, on the other hand, does not cause spontaneous pain but may restrict movement or cause muscle weakness. Someone experiencing muscular limitations may become aware of pain coming from a latent trigger point only when pressure is applied directly over the point. Both the active and latent trigger points will cause a localized twitch response when pressed or needled. Pressure on the trigger point may cause motor dysfunction of the affected muscle or an autonomic response such as sweating and dizziness. A local anesthetic can provide near immediate pain relief in treating a trigger point. One indication that you might have a myofascial pain syndrome is if you refer back to your avatar and note that you have X'ed discrete and localized areas of pain.

Myofascial pain syndrome is in fact closely associated with trigger points. More specifically, myofascial pain syndrome can also be defined as a set of symptoms experienced in the trigger points of an injured muscle bundle. Myofascial pain can be connected to other pain syndromes, such as headaches, temporomandibular joint dysfunction (commonly known as TMJ), and a variety of low back pain syndromes. If you suffer from myofascial pain syndrome, you're likely to have a decreased range of motion in your arms and legs, and altered posture, and you'll describe pain in a muscular area, but touching that area can, strangely, produce pain elsewhere in your body. Interestingly, the pattern of pain doesn't particularly follow the distribution of a local nerve, and doesn't necessarily follow the distribution of one of the nerve roots. This is what makes trigger points so unique, and the subject of Dr. Travell's books and manuals, which describe the patterns trigger points can make in the body.

From Dr. Travell's work, we now know that the most common trigger point locations in the low back include the gluteal muscles and those of the legs, including gastrocnemius (large calf muscle), hamstrings, and quadriceps. It's important to note that these areas may cause pain that radiates to a distant location.

Tender points, by comparison, are associated with pain at the site of touch only. Furthermore, unlike trigger points, which exist in a taut muscle band, tender points usually occur in symmetric locations in the body, they do not cause referred pain, and they do not have a twitch response. They occur in soft tissue and may be numerous.

Identifying trigger points is a skill learned by clinicians and can involve a variety of techniques. Although ultrasound, electromyography, thermography, and even muscle biopsies have been studied, there is no laboratory test for the presence of trigger points. A trigger point may be felt as a rolling tight area under the fingertips, and where pain is experienced when pressure is applied. Another way to identify trigger points is by tapping or needling the point to produce a twitch response. These remedies aim to control myofascial pain but can require multiple treatments. Treating trigger points can also reveal other points and sources of muscle strain.

As you can imagine, trigger point injections entail the administration of a local anesthetic—and sometimes a corticosteroid as well—into one or more trigger points, using a needle. With the injection, the trigger point is made inactive and the pain is alleviated. Trigger point injections are used to treat many muscle groups, not only the lower back and neck. They are frequently done in the arms and legs. In addition, they can be used to treat fibromyalgia and tension headaches. People who suffer from myofascial pain syndrome and who don't respond to other treatments often try trigger point injections. Note, however, that the effectiveness of trigger point injections for treating myofascial pain is still under study.

I can rarely predict which patient will benefit and for how long, but the risks of the procedure are so low that I include it in my armamentarium of resources and techniques and reserve its use for those patients whose avatars are consistent with the diagnosis. These factors mean, however, that it is unlikely that we will ever have good evidence as to its efficacy. The nature of the procedure makes it ripe for overuse, although, with few risks and side effects, it may be to the patient's ultimate advantage.

EPIDURAL STEROIDS

I would venture to say that there is hardly a patient I see who has not had a trial of epidural steroids. I found this to be the case, no matter what the diagnosis! The conditions for which patients have received epidural steroid injections include an acute herniated disc, spondylolisthesis, chronic low back pain, and spinal stenosis, among others. This in itself raised a red flag in my mind because I could think of few other treatment options used as often for so many different diagnoses. Only aspirin, acetaminophen, or possibly non-steroidal anti-inflammatories have been used as widely.

In fact, lumbar epidural steroid injections are so common that they seem to have become the standard of care. My clinical observation was corroborated in the Spine Patient Outcomes Research Trial (SPORT) randomized controlled trial on the treatment of lumbar disc herniations. In that trial, 42 percent of largely middle-aged subjects had an epidural steroid injection prior to enrollment in the study, and 56 percent of the individuals who underwent nonoperative therapy in that trial had an injection over the course of the study. And among all the patients receiving treatment for spinal stenosis in the degenerative spondylolisthesis branch of SPORT, 55 percent had an epidural injection prior to enrolling in the study and 45 percent of those receiving nonoperative treatment had an epidural steroid injection during the study. In 2007, a systematic review by the American Academy of Neurology, led by Dr. Carmel Armon, found little evidence that epidural steroid injections had a positive long-term impact on patients with radicular pain. The review concluded that epidural steroid injections did not improve function, did not reduce the need for surgery, and did not provide long-term care. Similar findings were reported by a group of doctors in the Netherlands led by Dr. Pim A. J. Luijsterburg in 2007.

In one article that I found particularly upsetting, Dr. Richard Deyo commented that the use of epidural steroids, and spinal injections in general, "may reflect financial incentives in that performing injections pays better per unit of time than talking to patients or performing other types of non-invasive therapy." It has also been suggested that a rise in the number of ambulatory surgery centers may play a role in the proliferation of these types of injections. In an article published in *Spine* in 2007 titled "Increases in Lumbosacral Injections in the Medicare Population," Dr. Janna Friedly of the University of Washington suggested that a rise in the number of outpatient surgery centers (where you have same-day surgery that does not require an overnight hospital stay) also may have played a role in the proliferation of injections. She rightly said, "Clearly physicians with ownership interests in ambulatory surgery centers may have direct financial incentives to perform more procedures." Her data suggested that from 1995 to 2005, the percentage of injections being performed at ambulatory surgery centers increased from 13 percent to 28 percent. While I find Dr. Deyo's and Dr. Friedly's comments and conclusions disturb ing, I must admit that I too have come to similar conclusions without the benefit of these large studies.

This is an unfortunate commentary on the way we practice medicine, and it warrants attention because it's an important lesson for you, the patient, to be vigilant and questioning when it is recommended that you undergo a trial of epidural steroids or, as I discussed in another part of this book, facet injections. I do, however, want to add that these issues are not so black-and-white. While randomized clinical trials frequently do not support the use of these treatment modalities, as is also the case of kyphoplasty or vertebroplasty, you already know that such techniques can have remarkable effects on some people. In addition to my own remarkable experience with a facet injection, I've had patients similarly respond very well to these options. On another, personal level is my wife's elderly uncle, who at the age of eighty-three was suffering from severe spinal stenosis and, because of a severe cardiac condition, was not a surgical candidate. My aunt and her husband called me and wanted to know what I thought of his undergoing a trial of epidural steroids. I reviewed the literature with them as I just reviewed it with you, and presented it in what I thought was a clear-cut and analytical manner. Yet their response was the same lament I hear from countless others: "What else is there to do?" And therein lies the dilemma.

Whereas even large randomized controlled studies would indicate no effectiveness for a specific trial, when it comes down to an individual patient—especially an elderly patient suffering mightily and with no other treatments are available—it's hard to say no. It's particularly difficult to shun such an option when the treatment is relatively non-invasive. My wife's uncle underwent the procedure and experienced a positive outcome, which lasted for many, many years.

Stories like this call to mind something I've noticed in the literature. At the end of many scientific articles, the authors—despite their own criticism of interventions such as epidural steroids—frequently point out that "this modality may be effective in a subgroup of patients, which requires further research." Statements like that make me want to tear out what little hair I still have left because on a practical level, as a practicing physician, it does not help me! I wish the literature reflected the reality of caring for patients in my office who have no other options but to try epidural steroids. They could fall into the majority of people who don't gain relief, but they could be part of the small minority that does.

The lesson here is that reviewing clinical trials won't necessarily help you decide whether or not epidural steroids are right for you. If you're among the "subgroup of patients" that responds well to the treatment, then it's for you. Until we have studies that can distinguish between those who will find relief from procedures such as epidural steroids, and those who will find them useless, we must be willing to experiment with them on an individual basis. So, if your doctor recommends them, by all means proceed with caution and keep your expectations in check, but know that they could work wonders on your pain. I also recommend that you ask your doctor about the latest technologies available to you that can help determine whether or not you're an ideal candidate for epidural steroids. As I briefly mentioned previously in chapter 5, while I was writing this book a new study emerged showing that certain proteins found in spinal fluid may point to who may benefit maximally from steroids. Wouldn't it be nice to know, before you try this method, if the proteins in your spinal fluid give a resounding green light? Remember, for updates to the latest studies, go to www.drjackstern.com.

Integrative Therapies

ACUPUNCTURE

There are more than thirty diseases or conditions for which acupuncture is recommended, according to the World Health Organization. But one of the main, most popular uses of acupuncture is for pain relief, and this method dates back centuries. Followers of Eastern medicine know that illness is often couched in terms of energy imbalances in the body. To activate a rebalancing and return the body to health, stainless steel needles are used to stimulate the body's fourteen major meridians, or energy-carrying channels. That may sound unscientific and difficult to prove, but because acupuncture targets points that are close to nerves, it is also believed to decrease pain by stimulating the release of endorphins—morphine-like chemicals that block pain.

Is there a role for acupuncture in the treatment of chronic low back pain? It appears so, although the type of acupuncture you receive might not matter. In a German study published in 2007 in the prestigious *JAMA Internal Medicine*, researchers compared a traditional form of Chinese acupuncture with a simulated but inauthentic acupuncture treatment consisting of a superficial needle at non-acupuncture sites. They also compared these results to a group undergoing conventional therapy, which consisted of a combination of drugs, physical therapy, and exercise. All of the participants underwent ten thirty-minute sessions twice a week for a total of five weeks. The researchers wanted to see how their participants fared after six months using what's called the Von Korff Chronic Pain Grade Questionnaire and the back-specific Hannover Functional Ability Questionnaire. These are questionnaires that help researchers determine the extent to which their participants responded to treatment.

The results were really quite amazing. Acupuncture clearly made a positive difference in the lives of people suffering from back pain, but the difference between the acupuncture groups—both real and "sham"—were minimal: 47.6 percent of those who underwent traditional acupuncture reported feeling back pain relief, while 44.2 percent of those who underwent the "sham" acupuncture reported feeling better, too. But the people who experienced conventional therapy didn't respond as strongly: only 27.4 percent of them showed improvement.

The authors concluded that acupuncture—even when it's not conventionally administered—proved to be twice as effective as conventional therapy. They also noted that this was the first time that acupuncture was demonstrated to be superior over conventional therapy. More studies need to be done to further flesh out this remarkable outcome, for this study had its limitations in some regards (one of them being the fact that it restricted the number of sessions to ten.) Nonetheless, it was enough to convince the German government to make acupuncture an insured benefit for chronic low back pain. For the first time, acupuncture was placed on an equal footing with conventional therapy for insurance purposes.

The fact that both the real (penetrating) and the fake (non-penetrating) forms of needle treatment had such a similar effect was surprising. It may be that the benefits of acupuncture have something to do with the way the body transmits or processes pain signals. Or it could be that the needles caused a "super-placebo" effect, triggering a real reaction in the brain that changes the way the body perceives and responds to pain. Regardless of how acupuncture helps relieve back pain from a biological standpoint, one thing is certain: Acupuncture, especially when it's of the conventional Eastern type, can provide significant relief and help people who respond to treatment require less pain medication.

Finding an acupuncturist is easier today than it used to be, simply because acupuncture has become much more common as a method of healing. It's nearly as simple as looking for a dentist. You could ask around and you'll probably find that friends have already been to one. You could look one up in the phone book or on the Internet. Online, you'll find that there are many and they are usually listed by city and state. Very often, your family doctor can give you a few leads, especially now that traditional medical professionals are referring cases to acupuncturists, and the line between the two streams isn't as rigid as it used to be. For all you know, you may just discover that your physician has done a course either in acupuncture or in an associated field.

Once you have a few names, research their credentials as you would any other health care professional. You could do this by checking to see if your state has training standards for acupuncturists. Not all do, but if yours does, it might be a good idea to find out a bit more about the professional you are considering. This is not to say that everyone with a certification is good, but it is an assurance of recognized training. You should expect an acupuncturist to look at your symptoms as any other health care professional would. However, if you are looking to one for a diagnosis of your ailment, you may be disappointed. Unless, of course, he or she is also a trained traditional medical practitioner.

Once the acupuncturist has an idea of the extent of your back pain, he or she will probably give you some idea of how much it will cost you. This will depend on the number of visits, and these in turn will depend on many factors, such as your age, your general state of health, the severity of your symptoms, and so on. There might be just one session needed, or on the other hand, you might need to keep going for weeks. You'll find that acupuncturists will cost less than physicians who also have training in acupuncture.

Does your insurance cover acupuncture? It may, but you will need to talk to your insurance carrier to be sure. You may also need a referral from your physician.

My take-home message: There is evidence that patients with low back pain benefit from acupuncture, but the studies can't say which patients will benefit and which specific set of symptoms will respond to acupuncture. This makes it challenging for me to know who to refer to the acupuncturist. One nonscientific criterion I use is whether the patient is open to this idea. And of course I make sure that the acupuncturist is experienced, skilled, and willing to communicate with me about the patient's progress.

ALEXANDER TECHNIQUE

I'm very familiar with this technique because my wife is a physical therapist and a longtime Alexander practitioner. The Alexander Technique emphasizes proper alignment of the head, neck, and spine so that the body can move more efficiently. The name comes from its developer, Shakespearean reciter Frederick Matthias Alexander, who developed the method at the turn of the twentieth century after concluding that poor posture was responsible for recurrent episodes of losing his voice. You'll want to find a practitioner who can guide you through these movements and teach you how to recognize and release habitual tension that interferes with good posture. The goal is to reduce muscle tension and restore the body's natural poise. The Alexander Technique works especially well for people who have postural problems or who suffer from chronic back pain and sciatica as a result of what I have been calling "misuse," which is probably the most common cause of low back pain. A study published in the *British Medical Journal* found that lessons in the technique helped patients with chronic back pain. A 2011 study published in *Human Movement Science* concluded that the Alexander Technique increased the responsiveness of muscles and reduced stiffness in patients with lower back pain. It can improve balance in older people, reduce depression, and improve function in people with Parkinson's disease. And there's anecdotal evidence to show that this approach can also aid people with arthritis and improve breathing, repetitive strain injuries, and stress-related disorders.

The Alexander Technique is typically taught in private, one-on-one sessions for thirty to sixty minutes at a time. Try one session to see if it's for you. If so, consider committing to ten lessons. Individual lessons cost $60 to $125, depending on the teacher's experience. Insurers will not likely reimburse you, so look into group lessons. The teacher will watch how you sit, stand, and walk, and help you to learn how to perform these movements on your own. You may find yourself on a padded bodywork table so that the teacher can gently move your head and limbs to release areas of tension. You might feel taller after your first session, as some report feeling as if they've gained some height due to the lengthening of the spine achieved by the technique. To locate an expert in this method near you, go to the American Society for the Alexander Technique at www.amsaton line.org.

My take-home message: I have had the greatest success with those patients whose pain is acute to chronic with no single identifiable pain generator and whose pain is postural and/or the result of repetitive misuse. Most patients will quickly know if they experience pain relief. The challenge is for them to integrate the newly learned pain-free status. And like all newly acquired skills, it takes a long-term commitment to have it become a habit.

FELDENKRAIS METHOD

Moshe Feldenkrais, a Russian-born physicist and athlete who wasn't satisfied about the fifty-fifty prospects of improving his debilitating injured knee with surgery, searched for another solution that led him to develop his own method for healing. His technique uses subtle movements to retrain the nervous system, which is the true source of perceived pain.

People who specialize in Feldenkrais guide clients in breaking down movement patterns, which are repeated with many variations, to reeducate the brain and nervous system to change patterns of movement. Through repetition, people experience new, more efficient ways of moving as "normal." Many candidates for the Alexander Technique are also candidates for this method. It's also been suggested for older individuals who want to maintain or increase their range of motion and flexibility. Because of its emphasis on enhancing overall mobility, this method has been shown to benefit people whose movement has been restricted by injury, stroke, fibromyalgia, cerebral palsy, and of course back pain and other disabling conditions.

I have very limited clinical experience with this technique and have not seen publications studying its use for low back pain. I have a number of friends and colleagues, however, who utilize the method as a means to move with less effort, and they find it makes daily life easier. As with many of the other techniques outlined in this chapter, you'll want to find an experienced practitioner of this method. Mastering this type of motion will require some step-by-step guidance, in either private, one-on-one sessions or group settings. To locate a practitioner in your area, go to the Feldenkrais Guild of North America's website at www.feldenkrais.com.

MASSAGE THERAPY

Earlier I told you about my own experience with back pain and how a massage therapist caused some serious pain and injury to my back. But don't get me wrong: There is a time and place for massage therapy in the treatment of back pain, and it shouldn't trigger harm. My injury was more or less an accident that would not have happened had I received a different type of massage with a more experienced masseuse. Allowing a large person to tread on your back should not be equated with "massage therapy."

How strong is the evidence on massage therapy as a treatment for chronic low back pain? The jury may still be out, but there's plenty of anecdotal and some mounting scientific evidence to consider. In 2007, Dr. Jennie Tsao at UCLA looked at massage as a treatment for chronic musculoskeletal pain in general, and then at chronic non-specific low back pain in particular. She found fairly robust support for the analgesic effects of massage therapy on chronic low back pain, but only moderate support for other types of pain, including shoulder, neck, and headache as well as in the treatment of fibromyalgia, mixed chronic pain conditions, and carpal tunnel syndrome. Dr. Tsao's data was based on a relatively small number of studies, however. In an earlier collaboration study performed in 2002 and led by Dr. Andrea Furlan, researchers also found the evidence somewhat limited, but good enough to suggest that massage therapy has positive effects on patients with chronic low back pain, particularly in terms of improving symptoms and function, and especially if the massage therapy is combined with exercise and education. Unfortunately, conclusions like these can meet opposition. Data coming from Europe and published in the "European Guidelines for the Management of Chronic Nonspecific Low Back Pain" in 2006 plainly stated that there's no reason to recommend massage therapy as a treatment.

Swinging the pendulum back the other way, then came a more recent study in 2011 that compared relaxation massage therapy to targeted deep tissue massage and "usual care"—medication and physical therapy. To be clear, targeted deep tissue massage is sometimes referred to as structural massage for its focus on specific pain-related issues, ligaments, and joints; myofascial pain release would be considered part of this category.

The study, published in the *Annals of Internal Medicine*, shows that relaxation massage is indeed an effective treatment for lower back pain. After ten weeks, the results were dramatic: Nearly two-thirds of the patients who received either type of weekly massage said their back pain was significantly improved or gone altogether. Only about one-third of patients receiving the usual care experienced similar relief. In some cases, researchers reported that the benefits of massage— whether of the relaxation or deep-tissue variety—lasted for six months or longer.

My take-home message: Until there is clear evidence one way or the other, each of us can choose to test these methods out. If they work, that's great. If they don't, you can move on to something else.

In my own experience, massage therapy has undoubtedly helped some of my patients. I can't usually tell from the get-go who might benefit from massage and who might not, and in almost all cases the pain relief is usually short-lived. So, if you have access to massage therapy, then there's no harm in seeing if this works for you so long as you find a well-qualified therapist who is experienced in working with back pain sufferers. To this end, I do recommend alerting your massage therapist to your back challenges so he or she can make appropriate modifications. And you never know: You just might find a therapist who can work on your back in ways that do in fact bring unprecedented relief.

SPINAL MANIPULATION

Spinal manipulation is another technique that's been around for centuries, arguably for as long as humans have tramped across earth searching for therapies to address pain. Today, spinal manipulation, which is the application of force to the spinal joints in hopes that it restores the spine's structural integrity and initiates the body's natural healing processes to reduce pain, is often used in combination with other forms of therapy, such as massage and exercise. There are several professions emphasizing and/or using manual therapy and spinal manipulation therapy (SMT), including chiropractic, osteopathy, and physical therapy. There is also a large body of evidence evaluating SMT in a number of existing systematic reviews. These reviews, however, come to different conclusions on the effectiveness of SMT for the treatment of low back pain.

Chiropractors often refer to manipulation of a spinal joint as an "adjustment." Because chiropractic receives a lot of attention in back pain circles, I'm going to focus on the subject here and share my thoughts. For the purpose of full disclosure, let me tell you that, unlike many colleagues of my generation, but fortunately not subsequent generations, I appreciate the role of chiropractic. I have sat on the

Board of the New York Chiropractic College and still sit on the New York State Board of Regents of the Professions for chiropractic.

Early in my surgical career, I encountered several patients who were neurologically intact, meaning they had normal sensation and strength in their muscles, but had significant low back pain and imaging studies consistent with a herniated disc. I also saw a larger number of patients with severe acute low back pain without radicular pain and whose CT and MRI scans didn't show a likely cause. The patients in both of these anecdotal groups improved significantly with chiropractic adjustment and in some cases avoided surgery altogether. Since that experience, I've actively collaborated with a significant number of chiropractors in devising treatment regimens for patients. But, having stated my bias, I also need to say that there are very few studies that actually show the efficacy of chiropractic or the efficacy of chiropractic as compared to other modalities.

In all fairness, the same comment could be made about most complementary medicine modalities. In an attempt to create some sense of this chaos, a group of researchers led by Dr. Daniel Cherkin in a Seattle-area HMO published a very interesting paper in the *New England Journal of Medicine* in 1998 that compared chiropractic manipulation with McKenzie exercises and a third group of patients who simply received an educational booklet on low back pain. This particular study excluded patients with radiating pain down the leg, and it lasted a month with a two-year follow-up. The researchers chose to examine the apparent benefits of chiropractic manipulation and McKenzie physical therapy because they are two of the most widely employed therapies.

Contrary to what you might think, Cherkin's group found that these methods are only marginally more effective than the educational booklet. Both therapies provided patients with slightly greater pain relief than the booklet, but neither of the treatments offered a significant *functional* benefit. There was no significant difference among the groups in a number of days of reduced activity or missed work, or in recurrences of back pain. The big differences between treatments? Patient satisfaction and cost. Fully two-thirds of the subjects in the therapy group rated their care as very good or excellent as compared with just 30 percent of the people in the booklet group. The high levels of patient satisfaction and slight reduction in symptoms associated with the two therapies came at a premium, however. It cost hundreds of dollars more to care for the physical therapy and chiropractic groups than those who just got the booklet.

The results of this study would lead you to believe that the McKenzie method of physical therapy and chiropractic manipulation are just not worth the extra money. But the results bring up a few good points.

First, the slight benefits attributed to the physical therapies could be the result of an "attention placebo effect" whereby the level of attention given to the patients receiving therapy changed their perception of pain. And second, the study was limited by the facts that it was sponsored by a civil health care system, lasted only one month, and excluded patients with sciatica. So perhaps the results would have been different under different circumstances.

In 2013, Dr. Christine Goertz and her colleagues at the Palmer Center for Chiropractic Research in Davenport, Iowa, conducted a randomized double-blind study that compared standard medical care alone with chiropractic manipulative therapy *combined* with standard medical care in men and women aged eighteen to thirty-five. The combined treatment showed a significant advantage for decreasing pain and improving physical functioning.

My take-home message: What a study like this does for me is provide some reassurance that if I had a choice between referring a new patient with the onset of low back pain—particularly someone without radicular symptoms—to her family physician or to her chiropractor, I would opt to send the patient for chiropractic treatment as well as to her physician.

BIOFEEDBACK

Later in this book, you'll get a better sense of why and how biofeedback can be so beneficial. At the center of this technique are identifying and learning how to change your brain's response to pain, which could help ease your back pain. This is very similar to how the Feldenkrais Method works.

As you've been learning, pain is really just a perception rooted in the brain. If you can gain control of or change the patterns in your brainwaves that occur in response to pain, you can effectively reduce your back pain. While this may sound a bit abstract, another way to look at this method is to consider it as simply a way of directing biological information from your body back to your brain so that a learning loop is created and you learn to control those parameters.

Historically, people used biofeedback methods to control muscle tension, skin temperature, and heart rate. Today it can be used for pain management, including back pain. Biofeedback techniques have not been thoroughly studied, so the data supporting their use in pain management are scarce. In a recent study of 128 adults with chronic back pain and significant disability, biofeedback was shown to be a possible complementary technique to psychological pain management training. A second study examining the use of biofeedback in headache pain found that biofeedback may be a good complement to relaxation techniques, but noted that biofeedback is a costly and lengthy process that does not appear to result in proportionate gains in pain management. That said, it should be noted that even though biofeedback may not necessarily directly reduce back pain for you, it can indirectly help by having a positive impact on reducing your overall stress, which exacerbates the pain.

When you visit a biofeedback specialist, you'll likely be connected to machines that monitor your brainwaves and vital signs, such as your heart rate and skin temperature. Biofeedback uses electronic instrumentation to monitor your body's specific, often unconscious physiological activities and habit patterns and then "feeds back" the information to you. Once you are aware of what your body is doing, you can change those patterns to reduce or eliminate your symptoms. While you undergo the biofeedback experience, you will be interacting with a visual of some sort that tells how your body is responding. This will help train you to control your body's responses.

If you choose to try biofeedback, you'll want to find a qualified practitioner. Look for someone who is certified by the Biofeedback Certification International Alliance (www.bcia.org), has many years of experience, and has a diverse background as a health practitioner. You may also want to consider your personal interaction with the professional you choose, since you'll likely spend several sessions with this person. Many people need about fifteen sessions to manage mild back pain and up to seventy sessions for chronic pain.

YOGA AND PILATES

Yoga has become so mainstream today that it barely needs explaining. I've had many patients benefit from a routine practice to keep their bodies strong and pain-free. And studies have shown that just one class a week can be an effective tool for relieving low back pain. Although there are many different types of yoga, some more rigorous than others, the practice in general aims to enhance the body's muscular strength and flexibility, which in turn can prevent and reduce back pain while boosting overall functionality. It also engages the mind and often involves certain breathing techniques to coincide with the movements. As a stress reducer, yoga further has an impact on the perception of pain.

What's great about yoga is that it can be done anywhere, since it doesn't require the use of machines. If you don't have a studio near you, you can stream videos or download a program online to learn various yoga practices and find one that works for you. Start with basic yoga (try a vinyasa flow level 1 class) and be sure to avoid any positions that seem to aggravate your back.

The Pilates Method is also a popular and intense form of strength training based on the idea that the abdominal and pelvic muscles are the body's power center. Unlike weight training, it does not isolate muscles. Pilates is done with an instructor at a health club or studio, using special machines (reformer Pilates) or on the floor (mat Pilates). Movements are slow and aim to engage the mind as well as the body.

Developed in the early twentieth century in Germany by Joseph Pilates, who was a physical-culturist born in Germany in 1883, the method has gained enormous popularity in the last decade alongside yoga. But it's not just for managing pain. Similar to yoga, the Pilates Method helps build strength and flexibility, and supports endurance and coordination in the legs, abdominals, arms, and back. This explains why it has gained recognition in both medical and fitness circles as a beneficial form of exercise to address an array of concerns, from back pain to excess fat. But there's a caveat to consider: Traditional Pilates, especially when done on the floor using a mat, involves an excess of motion for the spine, which can actually increase the risk of spinal fractures in some people. For this reason, many of the movements typical of Pilates are not recommended for those with osteoporosis and osteopenia. But this doesn't mean that everyone who has these conditions should avoid Pilates. It helps to find an expert Pilates instructor who can tailor a program to your needs, modifying certain movements so that you stand to benefit—not increase your risk for further problems.

Because balance and control play a large role in the Pilates repertoire, the technique is a whole-body experience that also targets the deep stabilizing muscles of the lower back, pelvis, and abdominals. All of these muscle groups help support the body—and back. This promotes good posture, decreasing your risk not only for back pain but for falling. You can find a certified Pilates instructor at www.ideafit.com, the online home to the world's largest association for fitness and wellness professionals. In fact, this site offers a directory you can use to find a variety of fitness professionals, classes, yoga studios, and gyms in your area. Just click on the "FitnessConnect" tab on the home page.

Dr. Paul Marshall, formerly of the University of Auckland and now at the University of Western Sydney, published one of the first papers on the comparison between Pilates and stationary cycling for treating back pain. Measured at baseline, the Pilates group had significantly less pain, but at the six-month mark the improvement didn't last. The weakness in the study, in my opinion, was that the Pilates lessons were given for only eight weeks.

Like so many other therapeutic practices, yoga and Pilates are intended to be long-term practices. To expect the positive results to last is no more reasonable than to expect the results of a medication to last once you've stopped taking it.

TAI CHI

Tai chi is a mind-body discipline that has been practiced for thousands of years in China, and is gaining popularity in the West as a way to relieve all sorts of pains, including those related to the back and neck. It is easy to associate tai chi with groups of people in parks or gyms moving slowly and deliberately in synchronization. These people are using the same tai chi principles and movements created in ancient China and still practiced all around the world as a healing exercise.

Large, clinical studies on the health benefits of tai chi are lacking, but many who practice it report heightened feelings of well-being along with a variety of other health benefits, including improved strength and flexibility, reduced pain, better balance, and sound sleep. A few studies are beginning to support some of these claims. Researchers are particularly interested in tai chi's potential for providing benefits for older adults. The National Center for Complementary and Alternative Medicine (NCCAM) and other agencies are funding a wide range of tai chi research studies. In August 2011, the journal *Complementary Therapies in Clinical Practice* published a review of the research to support tai chi, and confirmed what the anecdotal evidence had been saying for a long time: The physical benefits of tai chi include balance and muscle strength; relief from the pain of fibromyalgia, osteoarthritis, and rheumatoid arthritis; and a psychological boost. All of these play directly into the back pain equation. No doubt we'll need to amass more evidence in the future that's rooted in science, but I think the proof is already there to at least consider tai chi a potential ingredient in healing.

So, what exactly is tai chi? It's a type of low-impact, weight-bearing, aerobic exercise. It began as a martial art, but as it developed, it took on the purpose of enhancing physical and mental health. Practiced in a variety of styles, tai chi involves slow, gentle movements, deep breathing, and meditation. The meditation is sometimes called moving meditation, and some people believe that tai chi's health benefits are due to its improving the flow of energy through the body. Unlike many other types of aerobic exercise (such as running), tai chi does not involve any jarring motions that create impact on the spine.

What makes tai chi so universally embraceable is the fact that it's non-invasive, relatively inexpensive, and gentle on the spine. Furthermore, tai chi does not require any expensive equipment and can be practiced anywhere. But, once again, tai chi is a "practice" (i.e., it requires a long-term commitment and aims to enhance general well-being); it is not specifically for back pain relief. Although I cannot say for sure that tai chi can directly relieve back pain, I will make two observations:

1. I have never seen a patient who practices tai chi. My belief is that this and other long-term-committed practices are more preventative than curative.
2. I also believe that individuals who make a long-term commitment to any regular physical practice are also more likely to be taking better care of themselves in other realms (e.g., diet, sleep, exercise).

Should you choose to try tai chi, you can likely find group classes in your community.

CHI GONG

Sometimes written as "qigong" and pronounced "chee gong," this practice involves a series of postures and exercises, including slow, circular movements, regulated breathing, focused meditation, and self-massage. Although it's considered a separate practice from tai chi, the two share similar characteristics and features. Like tai chi, chi gong aims to train the mind to direct the body's energy, or chi, to any part of the body. Some believe that, when moved correctly, chi can bring your body to a natural state of balance. Chi gong is believed to relax the mind, muscles, tendons, joints, and inner organs, all of which helps to improve circulation, relieve stress and pain, and restore health.

There are a variety of chi gong styles, and they are classified as martial, medical, or spiritual. Some styles are gentler whereas others, such as kung fu, are more vigorous. Practiced widely in the clinics and hospitals of China, chi gong may have broad health benefits. Most of the studies conducted on this method are limited in scope, however. Many are small case studies conducted in China—not large, randomized, controlled trials reported in peer-reviewed English-language journals. One small pilot study showed fewer symptoms and improvement in function among patients with fibromyalgia who were practicing chi gong. Larger trials are needed to confirm the results.

For more information about chi gong, tai chi, and energy medicine, you can search more than 4,000 citations online at www.qigong institute.org/html/database.php.

My take-home message: My own experience with tai chi and chi gong is limited. Both modalities require great commitment and the benefits will not be seen for months. The patients who have incorporated these modalities are making lifestyle changes and frequently also opt for a weight-reduction program and the practice of meditation. The reduction in low back pain in those patients has been quite dramatic.

RELAXATION AND MEDITATION

If you are one of the many sufferers whose back pain is the result of muscular spasm, or strain or tension from mental stress, meditation may be the right therapy for you. Even if your pain has a structural cause, regular meditation could still be of great benefit once the immediate physical problem is dealt with. Meditation may help relax the patterns of muscular tension responsible for the problem in the first place, helping to prevent a recurrence.

It is well documented that regular meditation promotes feelings of mental clarity and peace. Medical research has confirmed that meditation can also improve physical health. It induces a state of deep relaxation, which many experts believe is superior to sleep in its ability to refresh and heal the mind and body. During meditation, both the heart rate and rate of breathing can decrease, and brain activity may alter to patterns seen only during very deep relaxation. Regular meditation may reduce high blood pressure and ease stress-related disorders. It can also have a beneficial effect on many other conditions, including chronic pain, muscular aches and pain, asthma, insomnia, heart disease, and other circulatory problems. Those who routinely practice meditation report that their emotional stability improves and their powers of concentration greatly increase. Addictions and patterns of negative behavior are more easily overcome.

You can meditate in any sitting posture that is comfortable and allows your back to be held straight. The most important consideration is that the room should be warm but well ventilated; spacious; and free from noise, bright lights, and other distractions. Breathe through the nose rather than the mouth whenever possible. Breathe deeply, but gently, using the abdomen rather than the chest. Your abdomen should swell as you breathe in and flatten when you breathe out. When you breathe like this, your chest should hardly move.

Most people find it helpful to concentrate on an object, such as the flame of a steadily burning candle, or to close their eyes and repeat a mantra of short words or a phrase in their heads. Some visualize a pleasant scene, perhaps a flowing river or a beach. Others focus on their regular, deep breathing. The key is to find what works for you. The aim of meditation is to free the mind from conscious control, to allow it to become empty. You have to learn to let go of conscious thoughts and anxieties and allow the deeper, calmer part of you to emerge. Inevitably your mind will wander. Accept this and do not become irritated by it. As soon as you are aware that this is happening, gently return your concentration to the present. With practice, you will gradually learn to redirect these meanderings almost without thought and your stream of meditation will be uninterrupted.

Take your time and try not to become frustrated if you feel you are not making progress. If you force yourself, you are no longer meditating. Some people find it helpful to learn the ropes of meditation by first using a guided mediation audio that may be purchased or downloaded online.

NATUROPATHIC CARE

I've chosen to end this chapter with some thoughts on naturopathic care, which isn't invasive at all and encompasses a broad spectrum of therapies. By definition, naturopathic medicine is a system of integrative medicine based on the theory that diseases, including pain, can be successfully treated or prevented without the use of drugs. At the heart of naturopathic medicine is attention to diet, exercise, and massage. Hence, when treating low back pain, a naturopathic physician may and will include acupuncture, physical activity, nutritional advice, relaxation training, and written back care education material.

Because naturopathic care is not a stand-alone treatment, its effectiveness is difficult to evaluate. But we do have some evidence to consider: A rather limited Canadian study of warehouse workers with low back pain of at least six months' duration (but not bad enough to prevent them from working) showed some benefit to this approach. The workers were randomly split into two groups, one that received a regimen of naturopathic care and another that underwent a regimen of physical therapy advice and was given a back care educational booklet. Both groups were allowed to maintain any pain medication and other therapies (e.g., massage, chiropractic, physical therapy) that they had been on before. The study demonstrated that naturopathy was cost-effective and those in the naturopathy group did have a statistically significant improvement in terms of quality-adjusted life years.

Because naturopathic physicians are not licensed in the state of New York, my own exposure is limited. They are, however, licensed in the adjacent state of Connecticut. Those patients whom I have seen who are already under the care of naturopathic physicians are for the most part suffering from very mild chronic low back pain. And in general, these patients tend to be very open to the use of complementary/integrative treatment modalities. My advice to you: If you fit this profile and your state licenses this form of medicine, you might want to consider this as a treatment option. Be mindful, however, that it's the combination of therapies that creates the naturopathic approach. Whether or not you engage the services of a licensed practitioner, if you choose to participate in the therapies commonly used in naturopathy, such as acupuncture, massage, tai chi, and changes in diet, then you are taking a naturopathic approach. It helps, however, to have the guidance of a licensed naturopathic physician in this field, should you want to maximize the potential benefits of this modality.

ACTION PLAN

- In general, the treatment ideas described in this chapter are best suited to patients with acute or chronic low back pain but with minimal radicular symptoms (shooting pain down the legs). Before embarking on a trial of any of these therapies, it is wise to have a conversation with a spine specialist first to determine if there is a structural reason for your pain. This is especially true if you demonstrate the "red flags" (see page 81).
- If it is recommended that you try one or more of these therapies, be willing to until you find one that is most effective in treating your pain.

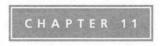

CHAPTER 11

The Trail from Acute to Chronic

The Psychology of Pain, Part I

P ERHAPS THERE'S no better way to illustrate the cascade of events that can occur when a person goes from a single, acute episode of back pain to becoming the chronic—and endlessly perplexing—patient than to hear the story of Jonathan D. His experience is emblematic of the challenges we face not just as doctors trying to heal our patients, but as human beings trying to maintain our quality of life when faced with a series of serious, unpredictable events that fuel relentless cycles of pain. Jonathan's plight also illustrates one of the most important aspects to understanding pain: the psychological underpinnings that can pervade in many cases.

When Psychological Pain Is
More Haunting Than Physical Pain

A new patient just getting started with me after a long and arduous journey, Jonathan wrote me an emotive recount of his personal story while I was putting this book together. I knew immediately that his experience was emblematic of the suffering and frustration experienced by millions of people. It was a call for help as much as it was a call for change in how we treat patients, and how we should come to define the word *disability*.

It all started on that fateful day of September 11, 2001. At the time, Jonathan was working at a large company located next to Grand Central Terminal in New York City. Jonathan was a crisis-management expert who found himself running up and down the granite staircase in Grand Central all day long. It was believed that the iconic station would be the next target for the terrorists who had already taken down the World Trade Center towers and a piece of the Pentagon in Washington, DC. At some point while climbing and descending all the stairs, Jonathan lost all power in his right leg. And although the nightmare of another terrorist attack thankfully didn't take place at Grand Central, a nightmare of a more personal nature did begin for Jonathan that day.

Jonathan is not the type of person you'd typically think would be vulnerable to an injury like this. Prior to 9/11, he was in great shape. He worked out about three to five times per week, jogged regularly, could bench-press 265 pounds, and was an active skier. A few days after 9/11, he returned to the gym and discovered that he could not even turn the pedals on the stationary bike without experiencing pain. By then he was walking with a severe limp due to the pain and went to see an orthopedic physician. Within two weeks of the injury he suffered a hernia on the right side of his groin (known as a right inguinal hernia to us doctors). Surgery for the hernia and recovery followed. In December he started physical therapy. Medical payments started to add up, and like so many others in his situation, he was advised to file paperwork with workers' compensation (WC).

It was clear that after several weeks of physical therapy, things were starting to get worse. His left knee began to ache in addition to his right, and the pain in his back flared up. Jonathan's injured right knee clearly was throwing off his body's mechanical balance, and now other parts of his body were under stress. Complications with his workers' comp case meant his right knee would not be operated on until the next summer, almost a full year after the original injury. And within that year, Jonathan had taken his fair share of falls, causing injury to his elbow, exacerbating pain in the left knee, and worsening the discomfort in his lower back. Naturally, his activity levels declined, which then had its own repercussions: His weight ballooned and his sense of well-being took a serious hit. It was also determined that his left knee would need surgery as well, but that wouldn't happen until 2004. Again, disagreements and bureaucratic red tape over the insurance payments caused the delay.

Jonathan stated it so candidly when he wrote:

After living with pain for so many years, you eventually end up accepting the lifestyle without really realizing it. In the past I have always healed from an injury and I expected the same from this one. A year goes by, then several more, and I keep thinking, "If I just work a little harder at it I can overcome it." Yet each year I am worse off than the prior. You start changing your daily activities in order to avoid pain or decrease the impact of the ongoing pain. You never think of yourself as disabled, but you just think of ways to avoid certain actions.

For Jonathan, pain became an everyday event. It infiltrated almost everything in his life. Walking or sitting for long periods of time hurt. If someone bumped into him at the market or he twisted slightly a certain way, the throbbing spasms would commence. Cold weather increased the intensity and frequency of his spasms, some of which were so excruciating that he'd yelp out loud like a wounded animal. Eventually his friends and family members got used to the new Jonathan and did their best not to worry.

There's no question that his relationships went through changes of their own. Jonathan had met his wife while on a ski trip, and they had always taken an annual trip out west to fulfill their passion for skiing. His son was just seven years old on 9/11, but Jonathan never skied with his family again and rarely participated in the kinds of sporty activities parents do with children, such as bike riding. An attempt to join his son's Boy Scout troop on an easy hike one day left Jonathan hobbling back to the car with his cane after going an embarrassingly short distance.

Every night Jonathan would lie on the floor to help relieve the pain in his back, which worsened during the day. He'd do whatever he could to manage the pain, from taking naps to applying heat or ice. As he put it: "These become normal activities, and again, you don't realize how much you have changed your lifestyle to deal with an injury."

Jonathan made a very insightful comment when he reached this point of the story. He asked: "At what point are you considered disabled? Is severe chronic pain a disability? Are severe spasms a disability? Is the constant modification of lifestyle a disability?"

Indeed, those are tough questions to answer. Jonathan's life had become a cycle of pain that went from borderline tolerable to totally intolerable and forced him to stay in bed for days on end. Jonathan had to learn which activities he needed to evict from his life forever, and which ones he had to modify in order to manage his pain. It took more than a dozen cycles of sudden, brief spasms for him to realize that he should no longer bend over to pull on his socks and tie his shoelaces; he'd have to find another way to achieve these tasks. Some things were virtually impossible to avoid, however. When a sneeze or coughing fit came on, Jonathan learned to brace his back against a wall to prevent it from jerking and triggering instant agony.

Of course there were other remedies that Jonathan picked up, some of which may not have been all that healthful. Alcohol, for example, became a daily habit that he realized needed to be curbed. So, he then tried a mix of other options, including exercise, more physical therapy, epidural steroids, more icing and resting, chiropractic care, and muscle stimulation. Soon enough, his days were consumed by focusing on trying to keep this incessant torment under control.

Not surprisingly, all of this meant that Jonathan could no longer do his job. His job required a lot of physical activities; on 9/11 he needed to be mobile and had to go up and down the stairs many times. Now he struggled on any staircase. At the time of his initial injury, and for several years afterward, Jonathan admits that he wasn't aware how severe or permanent his injuries were. He was now considered permanently disabled.

Today Jonathan has ongoing issues with both his legs and his back, plus in the past few years he has injured his neck during more than one fall. He fears that eventually he will be unable to walk, since over time this activity is becoming more difficult. Jonathan used to earn about $135,000 a year as a crisis manager; today he struggles to make $45,000 as a consultant. As Jonathan so poignantly explains:

> The devastating effect of a long-term disability is more than just physical and emotional. It destroys a person's livelihood. Unable to do my old job, I retrained myself in a new career that took me away from having to manage a crisis in a skyscraper. The new job involved driving to offices, spending several hours in a car, giving two- to five-hour presentations, often standing in front of a class, and then driving back home. At least I was avoiding my biggest nemesis, stairs.
>
> My chiropractor and others had warned me that my new

job's physical demands (i.e., long drives and standing for long periods of time) could aggravate my back problems, but I needed to pay the bills and put food on the table for my family. As the back pain increased I pushed on. I believe in working hard and I would deal with the pain later. Soon I had to limit my driving to every other day, then two days a week, and now I try to limit it to one day a month, due to the pain and spasms related to this activity.

Here's a man who went from being a strong, independent, and happy forty-two-year-old to being somewhat of an invalid, largely dependent on others, and clearly depressed. Everyday activities such as showering (and washing below the waistline), putting on socks and shoes, cutting toenails, and even pulling up underwear and pants are impossible for him to do by himself. Jonathan struggles to get up from a seated or reclined position. At night he sometimes uses both arms to lift himself on a banister to get up the stairs. He uses furniture, his cane, or other objects to help him when he changes positions. He continues to battle with his insurance company as the bills mount.

Is there a solution for someone like Jonathan? Can surgery help him? How could he have had a different experience, a better outcome? Where in this story did things go wrong?

There are a lot of issues that this story brings to light. For one, I wanted to share it because it paints a clear, albeit heartbreaking, picture of how the tides can quickly change. What starts as a seemingly minor injury morphs into a morass of ongoing problems and complications that affect every aspect of an individual's life. The difficulties entail not just the physical components but the deeply emotional, psychological, and even financial factors that play a commanding role in overall quality of life. Anyone who treats Jonathan at this point isn't dealing with just a purely physical or anatomical issue. There are a multitude of overlapping issues to address, most of which don't have direct and guaranteed "cures." In other words, there is no simple, hard-

and-fast set of steps, rules, surgeries, medication regimens, therapies, or exercises for Jonathan to follow in order to make a quick return to the person he was prior to 9/11. He will likely need to manage his pain for the rest of his life.

The obvious question is whether Jonathan's terrible condition could have been avoided. What if I had seen him soon after 9/11? Could I have changed his course? In all honesty, the adage that hindsight is twenty-twenty couldn't be truer than in this scenario. But I do believe that Jonathan's outcome could have been better if several factors had been different. The most apparent one was the sheer lack of a "captain"—a medical practitioner who knew Jonathan and whom Jonathan could rely on to coordinate his care and advocate on his behalf with the insurance company. This captain also could have helped him find the psychological support that he needed from the very beginning to deal not only with the pain but also his intense personal issues, educating him as to his legal rights under the workers' compensation rules. Jonathan could have further benefited from a spine specialist unaffiliated with any single type of treatment and who focused squarely on finding an accurate diagnosis initially and prescribing the appropriate treatment plan for Jonathan's particular symptoms. And this, as you know by now, is a task that this book undertakes.

Pain Perpetuating Pain

For years now, doctors like me have been trained to look for so-called yellow flags in a patient. I've already hinted at these in previous parts of this book, but now let's delve further into these as they stem from a story like Jonathan's. If there's one thing that his story demonstrates so well, it's the psychological toll that injury and unsuccessful treatment take on a person. And just as the physical aspect to injury can slowly evolve into myriad other physical problems, so too can the psychological aspect slowly shift from an initial nuisance or annoyance to profound feelings of depression, catastrophic thinking, anxiety, social withdrawal, so-called sickness behavior that has someone lying in bed all day, and a belief system that feeds the cycles of both pain and sadness. Jonathan has every right to lament that he's had a rough row through his recovery process, but for many people like Jonathan, something else begins to happen as their pain progresses without relief. The pain itself becomes the instigator and perpetuator of pain—the ultimate cause of interminable, untreatable misery. Let me explain.

Is It All in Your Head?

There's no question that the mind can play a definitive role in the instigation and progression of back pain. Pain, after all, is just a perception translated by none other than our invariably complex brains. In the next chapter I'll be taking you on what I hope to be a provocative tour of how sometimes we need to literally look above the neck to get to the bottom of back pain. We now have evidence that chronic pain alters the structure of the brain, leading to problems not only with pain signals but also memory, rational thinking, and the processing of emotions. How can pain be linked to our emotions? It's not as far-fetched as it may seem.

A 2006 study by a group of Northwestern University scientists led by Marwan N. Baliki, Ph.D., and A. Vania Apkarian, Ph.D., looked at areas of the brain involved in three pain states and found that sustained chronic pain, unlike acute pain, involves an "emotional-mentalizing" region of the brain. These researchers believe that continued activity in this region of the brain may help explain the psychological and behavioral costs of chronic back pain. In particular, they were able to uncover a few stunning new facts: (1) Chronic back pain is associated with a specific pattern of chemical changes in the brain, which is consistent with the loss of gray matter; (2) these changes account for decreased ability in emotional decision making; and (3) that this pattern plays a major role in chronic back pain. Indeed, it's a circular process—a vicious cycle. Dr. Baliki made a bold conclusion:

"These parameters account for over 70 to 80 percent of the variance for intensity and duration of chronic back pain. Therefore, they must be considered an integral part of chronic back pain." What Baliki is basically saying is that the extent to which you feel pain is directly related to physical changes in the brain, which in turn affect your emotional and sensorial experience to pain. So, it's not just physical changes in your back per se. I couldn't agree with him more.

Research like this begs the question: Can we find a way to treat the brain with drugs, which in turn treat the back pain? Researchers are currently trying to figure out this puzzle. In 2007, Northwestern University researchers attempted to come up with a drug treatment that could relieve the emotional component of chronic back pain. This is a totally different approach than the usual one of treating the sensory component to pain. The drug in question is D-cycloserine, which has been used to treat phobias. It works by improving attention and facilitating the end of acquired fear by altering activity in the prefrontal cortex of the brain. Researchers showed that this experimental drug greatly reduced the sensitivity of injured rats and the "protective" behavior that they would exhibit following their injury, and which would suggest the sensation of pain. The results were consistent with the idea that the drug relieved the emotional, rather than the sensory, component of pain. More remarkable than the onset of pain relief following an injection of the drug was the observation that the pain relief persisted for weeks. And the drug had no side effects.

How can this be explained? Put simply, we need to begin to think of chronic pain as the inability to turn off the *memory* of pain. The pain can start in a structural, anatomical area associated with the spine, but the pain fiber messages sensitize the central nervous system, so that over time the pain you feel becomes "automatic" and autonomous to some degree—separate from the initial structural problem. Another explanation for this is to consider pain's input from the body's other areas, which cause a generalized sensitization of the central nervous system. This implies that your experience of chronic low back pain does begin with a structural problem that involves pain messages traveling across pain fibers, but that the offending structural problem may be located in some other part of the body. You just happen to feel the pain in your back due to "mixed messages" on those pain fibers. And finally, it could very well be true that a key factor in your back pain is simply genetics, whereby you've inherited a heightened susceptibility to pain as well as a heightened vulnerability to the psychosocial traits that can contribute to endless cycles of pain. In fact, studies performed on fraternal twins suggest that disc degeneration (as measured by MRI scans) is strongly influenced by genetic factors. Surprisingly, genetics might trump environmental factors in the pain equation.

Such revelations have far-reaching possibilities as we begin to relieve what has clinically been the most difficult to treat: the suffering or the emotional aspect of pain. Historically, we've attempted to relieve chronic back pain by stopping the input of pain signals from the injured or dysfunctional part of the body. But what if the cognitive and emotional aspect to pain is the abnormal ingredient that's maintaining all the pain? Or that the remote control to our pain signals is stored in the brain—not the other parts of the body, despite apparent abnormalities? Those are questions that, as patients and doctors, we all need to ask ourselves. Future research will help determine if therapies like those proven in rats can work in humans (clinical trials on D-cycloserine in humans have yet to be completed). As you're about to find out in the next chapter, it will be a case in which we won't necessarily eradicate the pain, but will be able to change at least the experience of pain. You'll be aware of your pain, but its emotional consequences, and thus sensorial experience of pain, will decrease.

The studies that explore abnormal brain activity in people who cope poorly with back pain have been performed throughout the world—not just at places such as Northwestern University. In another study introduced in 2006, Gordon Findlay, M.D., of the Walton Centre for Neurology and Neurosurgery in Liverpool, England, presented results showing that patients who display abnormal pain behavior may have a distinctive pattern of brain activity in response to back pain and other painful stimuli.

The relationship between pain and the brain's physicality has also been borne out by research on people who suffer from hip pain. In a study published in 2010, Oxford University researchers found that chronic pain caused by hip osteoarthritis can actually shrink a brain region responsible for processing sensory cues and regulating consciousness and sleep! These researchers looked at gray-matter volume in a group of individuals before and after they got their hips replaced. Before surgery, the scientists compared the brains of patients who had severe hip pain with those of healthy, pain-free controls and found a significant loss of gray matter among the pain sufferers. But here was the unexpected finding: Nine months after hip replacement, the patients with hip pain had the same volume of gray matter as controlled subjects. So the good news is that the brain shrinkage appears to be reversed when hip pain is relieved—in this case, through joint replacement surgery.

I must add one more study to consider, which was published in the October 1, 2011, issue of *Spine*. This one had some intriguing findings related directly to back pain, underscoring the fact that back pain not only changes the brain but can also affect coordination. It's relatively common knowledge that our brains entail different regions and that specific areas of our brains control certain functions. What's probably not commonly known, however, is that every muscle in your body is controlled by specific areas of your brain. To accommodate complex movements in your body, the brain dedicates larger space for the more difficult tasks. The amount of brain space used for a specific muscle determines how coordinated that muscle will be. So the piano player will have a larger area of the brain devoted to controlling the muscles in the hands and fingers. A tennis player will have a larger area of the brain used for the muscles in the hands and feet to scoot deftly around the court and respond to balls.

When an Australian team of researchers led by Dr. Henry Tsao set out to understand to what degree recurrent back pain, even in young adults, could affect one's coordination, they must have been surprised by their discovery. They looked at the areas of the brain that control low back muscles and play a large role in low back/core stability. Specifically, Dr. Tsao's group examined these brain areas in people with and without recurrent low back pain, finding that in healthy individuals, these two muscle groups were controlled by two distinct areas of the brain. But in those suffering from recurrent back pain, a single area of the brain would begin controlling these two muscles, thus preventing the muscles from being used individually.

The results of this study show that recurrent low back pain is indeed accompanied by changes in the brain that cause a loss of coordination in low back muscles. The good news: Correcting the source of the pain and exercising these specific low back muscles can help restore coordination and break the cycle of recurrent pain.

The List of Yellow Flags to Look For

With these concepts in mind, let's turn back to you and your back pain. As I've been explaining, pain isn't just a sensorial experience. It also has its brain-based origins and shares a lot with our emotional experience. The movement from being in an acute state of pain to one that is chronic, as Jonathan's story exemplifies, is no doubt characterized by a rapid shift from a purely physical experience to a deeply emotional one. It helps to remember that acute back pain lasts fewer than three weeks; subacute back pain last-more than three weeks but less than three months; and chronic low back pain persists for longer than three months, or more than six episodes in twelve months. The alarming and disturbing statistic is that 90 percent of Social Security disability claims are caused by the 5 percent of patients who, like Jonathan, go on to develop chronic low back pain. The challenge for me and you is to prevent you from joining this elite group.

Only within the last decade or so have back pain specialists truly embraced the idea that back pain goes much further than anatomical sites. In 2010, one of my professional journals stated it perfectly: "The development of chronic disabling low back pain is more about psychology than anatomy. And patients with these risk factors may be more likely to respond to counseling, cognitive behavioral therapy, and exercise programs than they are to injections, interventional pain techniques, and lumbar surgery."

This new line of thinking is what led the American Medical Association to publish these so-called yellow flags that are predictive of which patients are more susceptible to the progression from acute to chronic pain. The hope is that the physicians will increase awareness of the yellow flags, and there will be early intervention to prevent this progression. What I find so fascinating with this new perspective is that the progression from acute to chronic low back pain is not necessarily a function of the type or degree of injury. It's also not a function of the patient's physical condition or other factors that one would logically associate with the development of pain—and the pain that becomes long standing and unresponsive to treatment. The study performed by investigators for the AMA confirmed what many of us, including myself, have long assumed: There are psychosocial indicators suggesting increased risk of progression to long-term distress, disability, and pain.

Let's look at the yellow flags. They were published in medical journals for professional readership, but I think it's imperative that you review them and ask yourself if any relate to you and your life. Fair warning: These yellow flags don't have a clear relationship to specific anatomic abnormalities in the back. But the evidence, according to a

THE YELLOW FLAGS

- Personal problems, ranging from financial difficulties to marital stress, etc.
- Low or depressed mood.
- Anxiety.
- Social withdrawal.
- A history of substance abuse.
- Problems at or dissatisfaction with your work.
- Your work includes heavy manual labor.
- A history of disability or other claims.
- Ongoing legal actions related to your health and insurance.
- Belief that your pain is harmful.
- Overprotective family or a lack of familial support.
- "Sickness behavior": You rest for extended periods, thinking that it will alleviate your pain.
- You're preoccupied with thoughts about your body, and you tend to have catastrophic thoughts.
- You consider yourself to be in poor general health.
- You consider yourself physically unfit.

careful systematic review and analysis of several studies performed throughout the world, is that the most important predictors of chronic disabling symptoms relate to psychological issues, problems with day-to-day function, and poor health. What we usually fail to treat are the other conditions that largely feed into one's back pain. And it is these conditions, or yellow flags, that we need to consider above all else.

Above is the list. Immediately, you see that these yellow flags relate to our attitudes and beliefs, emotions, behaviors, family, and workplace. Once again, I ask you to be totally honest with yourself and check off those issues that you can identify with.

What these yellow flags so clearly point out is that an individual's belief system about what happens and the fear about what happens can contribute to back pain. So just asking, "Gee, what do I think is going to happen to me with this back pain?" makes a difference. Or saying, "I won't get better, it's just going to get worse, my life is ruined, there's nothing I can do," can have unintended consequences on your psyche that ultimately set you up for failing treatment.

If you answered yes to most of these questions, you are at high risk for developing chronic low back pain. Even just a single yes response to any of these yellow flags indicates an increased risk for enduring a long battle with back pain. And once that happens, you're a member of an exclusive club of injured individuals who are in the fear-avoidance model of chronic pain. You quickly become reluctant to engage in activities and move your body, which leads to a loss of mobility and eventually disability and depression. We saw this progression in Jonathan. It can happen to anyone.

Just being aware of this vulnerability can give you the tools you need to intervene long before you become the chronic pain patient. Having the courage to notice and identify any yellow flags in your own life gives you a huge advantage toward back relief. The goal here is to stop the cascade of events—the vicious cycle—that can happen once an acute episode of back pain causes other problems to snowball, as they did for Jonathan. Use the strategies in the action plan below if you find yourself identifying with any of the yellow flags.

ACTION PLAN

If you've become a chronic pain patient and cannot find relief, and if the exercises in this chapter lead you to believe that some of the yellow flags reflect you, then I suggest the following:

- Ask your physician to refer you to someone who can administer what's called the Fear-Avoidance Beliefs Assessment Questionnaire. This actually entails four questionnaires:

- The pain-catastrophizing scale.
- Fear-of-pain questionnaire.
- Fear-of-avoidance belief questionnaire.
- The coping-strategy questionnaire.

These will give you a better idea of where you are emotionally and whether you are a candidate for several interventions that may help you. The most successful of those interventions include:

- Physical therapy and other activity-based interventions.
- Cognitive behavioral therapy.
- Intensive pain education and exposure intervention.

If you scored high on the questionnaire and are being treated by an individual pain management practitioner, you're probably not getting the best medical care. Likewise, if you're in a comprehensive or even multidisciplinary pain center that does not address the yellow flags, you're also not getting optimal medical care. That's because some of the key components of comprehensive intervention for a patient like you, who is at high risk for progression to chronic pain, need to include these four components:

- Physical therapy, including both individual and group exercise classes.
- Psychological therapy, including group and individual sessions as well as biofeedback.
- Occupational therapy.
- Case management that integrates the other components.

The challenge is that most physicians are reluctant or unaware of the psychosocial aspects of this disease, and many patients are afraid to answer the questions honestly for fear of being stigmatized with a diagnosis that will adversely affect their insurance and/or disability status. There are insurance providers who have been insufficiently educated to the benefits of these interventions and reimburse health care providers very poorly. My hope is that under the new Affordable Care Act rules, we as a nation will rectify this issue and change the way we approach back pain management so that there will be fewer patients who become chronic pain sufferers, and more who can reclaim a high quality of life.

CHAPTER 12

When It's Time to
Look Above the Neck

The Psychology of Pain, Part II

---

pain |pān|: *n.* an unpleasant sensory and emotional experience associated with actual or potential tissue damage, or described in terms of such damage.*

I'VE BEEN TALKING ABOUT PAIN since the first page of this book. It may seem odd to define it so precisely here now that we're so far into it, but we're going to look further at pain from a psychological perspective that really gives this definition justice. Indeed, pain is unpleasant and sensorial, and can certainly relate with actual tissue damage, but it's also something that can simply be "described in terms of such damage." What does this mean? Let's find out.

Pain is a wily adversary. Two different people suffering from ex-

---

* The International Association for the Study of Pain.

actly the same injury can experience the resulting discomfort in vastly different ways. In the definition of pain above, did you notice the word *potential*? And what about the reference to *emotional experience*? Is there more to physical pain than can be explained logically? As it turns out, yes. What goes on in our minds has more to do with pain than we ever imagined.

You'd think that with all of the latest technology and imaging capabilities we now have available it would be relatively easy to spot the exact source of pain and find a solution. But the research and statistics reveal a troubling fact: After undergoing the full range of diagnostic tests, 85 percent of patients suffering from low back pain still don't receive a precise diagnosis. The pain can't be pinpointed; there are just too many moving parts and a single pain generator cannot be identified.

On the flip side of this unfortunate fact is the disturbing disconnect between what imaging diagnostic tests may reveal and what's really going on within the human body. If an MRI, for instance, shows a herniated disc, you and your doctor may think you've located the culprit, but looks can be deceiving. You'll recall the 1994 study I described earlier that was published in the *New England Journal of Medicine*: When MRIs were done on the spinal regions of 98 people with no back pain or back-related problems, the doctors who examined the images but didn't know that the patients were not in pain found that 80 percent of the patients exhibited "serious problems," such as bulging, protruding, or herniated discs. In 38 percent of patients, the images showed multiple damaged discs. The relationship between disc degeneration and back pain becomes more pronounced with age; more than 80 percent of people over the age of sixty who don't have any back pain still demonstrate significant disc degeneration. These structural spinal abnormalities are often used to justify expensive treatments such as surgery, yet nobody would advocate surgery for people without pain.

Only young people have spines that look perfectly healthy. Degeneration is part of a normal process and it doesn't necessarily imply that their pain is a result of these changes. This is when we need to consider another pain generator that is largely responsible for a constellation of back pain cases but resides above your brow: the brain. It's the seventh pain generator, which deserves a whole chapter of its own. And, like pain, the brain can be just as much of a wily adversary.

A study published more recently in *Spine* pointed out similar findings to the *New England Journal of Medicine*'s 1994 study, and went a step further by integrating the psychological characteristics of patients. Dr. Eugene Carragee, a professor and vice chairman of orthopedic surgery at Stanford University School of Medicine, and his team followed a large group of patients over five years in an attempt to better understand the structural problems that cause chronic back pain. In addition to regular psychological evaluations, they performed MRIs and used discography (a diagnostic tool used to determine the structural integrity of an intervertebral disc) to examine the possible structural sources of back pain.

His results echoed what earlier studies were beginning to uncover: Neither discography nor imaging tests are necessarily reliable predictors of severe back pain. While two-thirds of patients with chronic pain had small fissures (tears) in their discs, 24 percent of patients *with no pain at all* also had the same damage. He raised an interesting question: Why do some people have a mild backache while others report crippling pain with the same findings on a variety of imaging studies?

When Dr. Carragee scrutinized the psychological evaluations of his patients, he concluded that a person's emotional state was better at predicting back pain than the person's anatomical condition. He found that the people who were best able to deal with their pain lacked certain mental and social risk factors, whereas those who harbored psychological challenges had a more difficult row and found their pain to be excruciating or, worse, catastrophic. Could this be the same phenomena we observed back in Step 1, when we looked at clusters of genetically similar people around the world who have categorically different experiences of back pain, yet whose pain levels should be relatively the same? How much of back pain is rooted in the brain and in one's social circumstances? To explore the answers to these questions, let me first tell you the story of Dr. O'Malley. His experience brilliantly demonstrates the power of the mind over the power of pain.

The Depressed Doctor with Chronic Back Pain

Every institution seems to have at least one outstanding doctor who is a master at diagnosing patients and who becomes a mentor of sorts for all the other doctors. Dr. O'Malley had this role at a hospital where I worked. When I first met him, he was someone who other doctors called upon whenever there was a difficult diagnosis to be made. It was also quite clear that for many of these same physicians, Dr. O'Malley was their own personal doctor. For a long time, I didn't have much contact with him, so I never got to know him very well. Then, one day out of the blue, he pulled me aside and asked if we could meet for lunch. By then he was about seventy-two years old, trim as ever in his well-tailored suits.

Surprised by his invitation, I assumed that he had low back pain because I'd noticed him in our office on more than one occasion seeing a colleague. During lunch, he went on to tell me that a lifting injury years ago had left him with chronic back pain. He treated himself with non-steroidal anti-inflammatory medication and changed his activities until the pain went away. But then the pain would return, and soon enough the bouts of pain overtook his pain-free periods. His episodes of pain grew more frequent and more painful. He was now experiencing pain all the time and it would sometimes radiate into his buttocks. Making matters worse, medications didn't help, and the examinations he'd had over the years never revealed a specific cause for his pain.

Dr. O'Malley approached me because he wanted to consider epi-dural steroid injections and facet injections. After all, he said, "I don't want to end up like my father." His timing couldn't have been more perfect. I was doing an extensive review of the scientific literature in preparation for writing this book, and a light went on in my head. I proceeded to do what other physicians hadn't done yet: take inventory of this man's psychosocial circumstances. It was clear that my colleagues had avoided this important task because we all respected this physician too much to probe his into personal life.

Over many such lunches over many months, which I began to refer to as my "Tuesdays with O'Malley," I became very attached to this man. I learned that his father was a laborer who had come to the United States from Ireland and ended his days in a wheelchair from what appeared to be spinal stenosis. Dr. O'Malley was a proud man who worked summers in order to afford medical school and was now "unwilling to give in to the pain." His wife was ill and they had no children, so he was her primary caregiver. He had no hobbies and didn't participate in sports because "medicine is my life." He had issues about retirement, and it was clearly evident that his own mortality hung over him. I am not a psychiatrist, but I didn't have to be one in order to realize Dr. O'Malley was depressed about his personal life, as well as depressed about the prospects for his future and the future of his chosen profession.

Eventually, over the course of our conversations, I suggested that his back pain might have some of its origins in places other than his back. Although he was skeptical, he was willing to listen and learn. We talked at length about the impact of depression on pain. I enjoyed his candor and openness about his personal life, which he explained was filled with fears—fear that he'd end up in a wheelchair like his father and fear that he wouldn't be able to care for his wife. We discussed the possible genetic and biochemical aspects of his pain, the yellow flags in relation to his attitude toward his work, and so much more. Dr. O'Malley ultimately decided to retire. He now lives in a warmer climate, and has time to exercise daily and care for his wife. He also sought counseling, which has been very helpful in his personal pain management. Although he wouldn't find total relief, his retirement helped him tone down the volume of his pain immensely so that he could continue to lead a very productive, satisfying life.

Retirement is not the answer for most of us, but Dr. O'Malley's story brings up several good points. Here was a man—a doctor—who was able to put aside his skepticism and look at his physical pain in a new light. He was able to appreciate that pain is often a physical manifestation but can take on a life of its own, one that can affect all aspects of an individual's life. And he was able to have the courage to address pain in "untraditional" ways by honoring his psychological needs and emotional health.

Searching for Proof of Cause

For centuries, the standard model of pain care has been to treat the pain by fixing the underlying abnormality, under the assumption that bodily pain is a response to bodily injury. Our back aches because a disc is bulging or a muscle is pulled. Fix the anatomical problem and the pain subsides.

But the reality is that pain is much more complicated.

Dr. John Sarno was among the first physicians to consider the psychological aspects to chronic pain. His seminal book *Healing Back Pain*, published more than twenty years ago, is still a best seller. It continues to stir controversy because back pain sufferers don't want to accept the notion of a psychosomatic component to their pain—code word for "you're crazy." Because we feel genuine physical pain, we expect pain to have a real and tangible cause rather than an ethereal one tied to our emotions or feelings. The key is to remember that even if your pain is caused by your mind, it doesn't mean it's not real and not painful. It just means that you have to change something in your mind—not only in your back. Since Sarno's bold theory first emerged, a growing body of evidence proves that, indeed, signals from the body can be distorted by the brain and result in real pain that has nothing to do, per se, with a structural injury or abnormality.

One of the first studies to highlight psychological factors in back pain came from a look at thousands of Boeing employees over a four-year period in the 1980s. During this time, about 10 percent of Boeing's people reported chronic back pain, and when doctors evaluated the factors that predicted the onset of these individuals' pain, they realized that structural back problems weren't the true cause. The workers who often lifted heavy objects were no more likely to experience disabling pain than those who had office jobs. As Stanford's Dr. Eugene Carragee later found, the best predictor of chronic pain was emotional distress. Those who were depressed or stressed out were much more likely to suffer from back pain.

In recent years, the medical community has finally started to embrace this other dimension to pain, which also means that one of the most powerful ways to treat chronic back pain—or any pain—is by treating the mind. When patients are taught how to deal more effectively with the negative emotions that accompany chronic pain, they often experience dramatic physical improvements.

Robert Kerns, Ph.D., has been studying the psychology of pain for more than three decades. Today he is a professor of psychiatry, of neurology and of psychology at Yale University. As a graduate student in the seventies, he first noticed a connection between pain and the brain. His early observation occurred when he treated a woman with serious back pain as a result of kidney disease. Despite the gravity of her physical condition, psychological therapy helped her cope with the pain.

Flash forward thirty-odd years, when Dr. Kerns continues to hunt down clues to all the anecdotal evidence he'd been collecting since the seventies. His 2007 study, published in *Health Psychology*, is perhaps his most definitive to date. After analyzing twenty-two trials that looked at the effectiveness of psychological treatments for patients with chronic low back pain, Dr. Kerns confirmed what he'd long thought to be true: Psychological therapy can alleviate pain. Patients with chronic back pain could diminish their hurt by simply learning how to think differently about their pain. The two particularly effective psychological interventions were cognitive behavioral therapy and so-called self-regulatory therapies, such as biofeedback. These therapies are not about addressing the physical pain, but rather shifting the patient's mental *perception* of that pain. It's amazing to think that routine medical care failed to provide substantial relief, whereas just a series of psychological treatment sessions that taught patients how to think about their pain could heal their hurt.

One reason why psychological interventions can be so therapeutic is that they teach patients how to develop strategies that make them feel better. Because patients often feel powerless and at the mercy of a seemingly illogical pain, they surrender to a sense of hopelessness that further exacerbates their pain.

As noted earlier, some of the most breathtaking research of late has come from Northwestern University, where researchers have discovered that pain can actually cause brain damage—more specifically, for each year people suffer from pain, they lose about a cubic centimeter of gray matter. And, over time, that brain loss adds up. Moreover, they've found that chronic pain, unlike acute pain, activates brain regions typically associated with negative emotions.

No doubt this kind of scientific finding is disheartening. People don't want to be told that their pain is programmed into their brains and embedded in their bodies like an intangible part that cannot be easily touched and fixed as could a herniated disc or torn muscle. There is hope, though. As I pointed out previously, scientists are currently working on treatments that might ease the suffering at its neural source using drugs such as D-cycloserine, which has been noted to significantly lower chronic pain in rats. While D-cycloserine was originally designed to fight tuberculosis infections, it also appears to turn the volume down on the emotional aspect of chronic pain. After thirty days of drug treatment, the rats didn't act like they were in pain. The hope is that when applied to humans, individuals suffering from chronic pain won't be bothered by the pain anymore even though they still have it. In other words, the pain will not necessarily be totally gone, but its emotional consequences and the resulting experience of pain's sensation will have decreased.

How is this possible? How can you have pain but not be bothered by it? It sounds counterintuitive and oxymoronic. In searching for a logical answer, it helps to understand that pain has two pathways—not one.

Pain's Two Separate Highways

When you fall down and scrape your knee, you feel the pain as pain receptors in your knee react to the injury and send a message immediately to your brain. That's one type of pain, and its pathway from knee to brain is clear. The hurt also has an obvious cause—the cut knee. But there's another pathway that is a much more recent scientific discovery and isn't based on signals from the body. We in the scientific community came across this other type when we identified a group of people who weren't bothered by pain after a brain injury. They still felt the pain and could accurately describe its location and intensity, but didn't seem to mind it at all. In other words, the pain wasn't painful.

What explains this? Turns out that these people's brain injuries involve an area of the brain that's responsible for processing emotions. So, they can't experience the negative feelings that normally come with painful sensations. Which suggests that our *emotions* about pain might be more influential than the pain sensation itself. Remove the emotion, and the scraped knee isn't so terrible.

This second type of pain, whereby the brain can't stop producing negative emotions associated with the painful sensations, is what often characterizes chronic pain. And such negative emotions can go on endlessly, even once the reason for the pain is gone. Although doctors have traditionally treated chronic pain as they would the first type of pain, hence the use of strong painkillers and surgery, now doctors like me are trying to take into consideration the second half of the problem here: the emotional underpinnings of ongoing pain. If we don't treat the emotional pathway, we probably can't remedy the chronic pain.

Persistent Pain Rooted in Emotions

Scientists have yet to find the exact mechanisms that link psychological problems to chronic pain, but the clues keep accumulating. It has been suggested that mental disorders can make people more likely to experience pain because certain regions of their brain and its innate neurotransmitters are affected by the disorder to change how they perceive pain. A brain-imaging study published by researchers at the University of Wisconsin–Madison in 2011 found that people with clinical depression were much less able to control their negative emotions. Not only could they not turn off their emotions, but the more they tried, the more they activated the areas of their brain responsible for emotion. So negative feelings beget more negative feelings. The Wisconsin researchers went so far as to suggest that depressed individuals might have a "broken link" in the brain, making it impossible to control negative emotion. Such cutting-edge research opens up new possibilities for treating chronic pain. In recent years, for example, other physicians and I have found that antidepressants, especially tricyclics, can be effective treatments for chronic back pain when an anatomical pain generator is not identified. These drugs help control the emotions that the patients cannot and, in turn, treat the malfunctioning of pain's second pathway.

Stress is yet another risk factor for chronic pain, and in many ways is just another angle to the emotional aspect of pain. I've had many patients, for example, who develop back pain during stressful periods in their life, such as the death of a loved one or after a job loss. And we now have some evidence that stress may affect the experience of pain. Joyce DeLeo, Ph.D., a neuroscientist at the Geisel School of Medicine at Dartmouth, found that chronic pain is often set off by a response from the immune system. DeLeo experimented with mice that were missing a specific type of immune receptor, showing that the mice were less susceptible to pain's persisting effects. Indeed, we've known for a long time that stress can profoundly change the nature of the immune system's response, but only now have we begun to map the connection between emotional stress and physical pain.

The emotional component to pain can be very difficult to measure and address successfully. In my own practice, I am very aware of my patients' psychological conditions prior to considering any kind of treatment, especially surgery. I see the impact of psychological issues in patients' experience of pain every day, and I am often left wondering whether there's a psychological substratum to their pain aside from, or in addition to, any structural abnormalities causing real pain. I've seen many chronic back pain sufferers who have a history of abuse, sleep disorders, post-traumatic stress disorder, alcoholism, substance abuse, depression, and other mood disorders such as bipolar disorder, postpartum depression, and premenstrual syndrome—all of which can encompass deep psychological elements that complicate their case.

I've even noticed a vast difference in the outcomes of patients who, for whatever reason, can't allow themselves to be pain-free, can't allow themselves the luxury of getting better, or who may get a secondary gain from their pain without even realizing it. Take, for example, the patient whose back pain originated in a car accident or at work while lifting heavy boxes. On a conscious or subconscious level, these patients know that their success in a lawsuit could be affected if they looked and acted in pain than if they entered the courtroom healed and happy. The man who gets injured at work and lives on disability may fear going back to work following a painful injury, even though his injury has healed. In this case, holding on to that pain can cause it to shift from a physically rooted (sensory) pain to an emotional pain that's sustained by pain's second pathway, and this can happen quite automatically and even below the person's conscious radar. I want to stress that it's not an act of malingering. Much to the contrary, it's a complicated web of physiological, emotional, and psychological aspects, none of which is clear-cut or easy to remedy.

Ghostly Lessons

The power of the brain in triggering illogical pain can be illustrated by the phantom limb syndrome—the perception of sensations, usually including pain, in an arm or leg after the limb has been amputated. To grasp the latest understanding of this phenomenon, it helps to turn to the studies of Dr. V. S. Ramachandran, who is director of the Center for Brain and Cognition and professor with the Psychology Department and Neurosciences Program at the University of California–San Diego. His innovative studies explore many of the uncharted depths in our understanding of how our bodies and brains relate to each other, often revealing unexpectedly complex processes for recognizing our physical selves.

In one of Ramachandran's most astonishing experiments, which was brilliantly reported by Robert Krulwich and Jad Abumrad for National Public Radio in 2009, he cured a patient's pain in a phantom arm through an illusionary trick of the eye. That's right: an optical illusion. His patient was complaining of excruciating cramping in his phantom arm due to a clenched (phantom) hand. In fact, his patient said that his "hand" was clenched so tightly that he could feel his fingernails digging into his "palm." To be clear, this patient was not delusional. He was well aware of the fact that his arm had been amputated and that the pain was throbbing from a nonexistent limb. "Yet his grasp of this reality was no match for his perceived pain," Kruluwich and Abumrad explain.

Dr. Ramachandran conceived an unusual treatment. As perfectly described by Kruluwich and Abumrad:

"He placed a mirror in a cardboard box and instructed the patient to place his existing hand inside the box, next to the mirror. When the patient looked down at the mirror, the reflection of his existing hand stood in as a visual replacement of his phantom limb. The patient was told to imagine that the reflection was in fact the lost limb, and to practice clenching and unclenching his hand while looking in the mirror.

"To the patient's—and Ramachandran's—surprise, the illusion worked. After two weeks, the patient's pain vanished, along with his perception of a phantom arm. Just how can a limb that no longer exists 'feel' pain? And why do some phantom limb sufferers gain relief from a low-tech optical illusion that tricks their brains into believing something that they already know?

"Clearly, the body and the brain are intricately involved in the perception of the physical self. But when sensory experiences don't match the brain's perceptions, how is this difference reconciled, and what can we learn from the disconnect?"

Dr. Ramachandran offers a useful analogy: He explains that the entire body can be thought of as a type of phantom. As such, the brain can interpret our sensory experiences as we interact with our environment. "The sensation of phantom limbs, and the experiences of patients who are able to relearn the way their brains perceive these phantoms, raise a host of fascinating questions," Kruluwich and Abumrad explain. "Neither purely physical explanations (that the irritation of severed nerves causes phantom feelings) nor purely psychological explanations (that feeling a phantom limb is a form of mental denial) can fully explain what patients describe.

"Instead, Ramachandran believes that a complex interaction between the physical and the mental is at play. The brain must reconcile the physical experiences of the body with the mental image, or cortical map, it has of the body. And as the body changes, this mental image can also be remapped."

But when the mental image doesn't follow the change in the body, that's how you can end up feeling pain in an arm that isn't really there. And with a mirror and a lot of creative thinking, Dr. Ramachandran was able to trick the brain into remapping its mental image. He calls this a "successful amputation of a phantom limb."

Despite the large body of evidence demonstrating the psychological component of chronic back pain, the vast majority of patients can't accept any diagnosis that involves their psychology. Not only do patients feel that they aren't being taken seriously, but they feel that such a diagnosis is offensive. It's like telling someone that he is insane, or that his pain is "all in his head." But as I stated earlier, the inability to identify a specific pain generator doesn't make your pain less real or less painful. It's simply an indication that you may have exhausted the search for culprits in your anatomical back and it's time to look instead at what's going on in the complicated network of your psyche and mind.

Treating Above the Neck

The good news is that while we can't always give birth to a brand-new back by realigning our spines or perfectly fixing our ruptured discs, we can control our perception of chronic pain. With the proper training, we can alleviate our own suffering and become our own best painkiller. Look no further than a study performed by Sean Mackey, M.D., Ph.D., to see this in action. Dr. Mackey is a professor of neurology at Stanford University and director of the Pain Management Center. He used real-time fMRI brain imaging to teach people with chronic pain how to control their conscious response to the pain using pleasant thoughts, mantras, or calming music. And all of them could see the direct impact of these strategies as they witnessed parts of their brains associated with chronic pain wane in activity. Most of them reported an average decrease in pain intensity by a significant 64 percent. Now that they could focus on controlling the pain, in their minds they were no longer at the mercy of a structural problem.

COMMON THERAPIES FOR TREATING PAIN ROOTED IN THE MIND

So, what can you do and where should you start? Following is a list of ideas to consider from top to bottom—from least to most invasive—in searching for your cure if traditional medical treatment hasn't done much and you suspect that you may have your brain to blame. (Some of these mind-body treatments were covered earlier, so refer back to them for more details on any of these therapies.) Speak to your doctor about referrals to professionals who specialize in these techniques, and ask your friends and coworkers for their recommendations as well.

Biofeedback

As noted earlier, self-regulatory therapies teach people how to take back control of their bodies. By giving patients information about their own internal processes (e.g., readouts of their blood pressure and brainwaves), the therapy teaches them how to modulate these processes. For example, you could be hooked up to a monitor that shows you your body's positions so that you know which position is painful and which is not. This interaction tells your brain to avoid the painful positions. Earlier I said that there are really no definitive studies proving that biofeedback is effective. A review of the research, which is this, shows that while biofeedback can be effective—especially for those who use it in combination with other therapies—it should be considered as part of an interdisciplinary pain management program. This is one of those cases in which, regardless of the scientific proof, if it works for you, it works for you.

Cognitive Behavioral Therapy (CBT)

A popular form of talk therapy, cognitive behavioral therapy teaches patients how to adopt a problem-solving approach to their pain. The simple premise of the treatment is that we are capable of controlling our own thoughts, emotions, and experiences. Therapists teach patients specific mental exercises, such as keeping a journal or practicing relaxation techniques, that help them manage their negative feelings and alleviate their suffering. As with biofeedback, CBT works best when used in conjunction with other pain management therapies. CBT has been well studied as an additive approach to traditional medical management of chronic pain. To date, the scientific literature supports the use of CBT with chronic pain to produce modest improvements in pain, fatigue, physical functioning, and mood.

Hypnosis

Unfortunately, hypnosis is a greatly misunderstood process. The common perception is that it's some type of quasi-magical procedure used effectively in the entertainment business rather than a bona fide medical procedure. This is hardly the case. Hypnosis is one of the oldest and most documented psychological interventions for reducing pain and suffering. Technically, hypnosis is the science of accessing and addressing repressed memories and thoughts that are causing subconscious angst and conscious physical pain. When a patient is placed into an altered state of consciousness (a state of deep relaxation), he or she can then be led to respond differently to pain messages. In the past twenty years, hypnosis has increasingly become an adjunctive therapy in the management of pain, as it has been shown to be effective in reducing both clinical and experimental pain.

The Alexander Technique, Chiropractic Medicine, and the Feldenkrais Method

Though these practices involve physical components, they have been used to help treat back pain rooted in the psychological mind. Please refer to chapter 10 for details on each of these integrative treatments.

Antidepressants

Antidepressants can be effective in the treatment of chronic pain. It's not clear why, but as I've mentioned, depression is a significant risk factor for back pain. What's more, if the pain has created depression, and you can treat the depression, you may be able to treat the pain. In other words, the depression is the avenue through which the pain is being sustained.

Anticonvulsants

If someone has pain, it may be an indication that there is abnormal regeneration of nerves. The nerves become agitated, causing a perception of pain, and anticonvulsants may help alleviate this reaction.

BELOW ARE ADDITIONAL methods that may seem to have nothing to do with easing pain that's rooted in the mind, yet these treatments can indeed help individuals who cannot otherwise relieve their pain, no matter where it's coming from.

Topical Creams and Oral Opiates

Sometimes a topical lidocaine can help, or even an oral painkiller. When it comes to ingested medications, however, the challenge is to find a balance between pain relief and side effects. Common painkillers such as Percocet and Vicodin do not come without their fair share of potential side effects, including chronic constipation, sleepiness, loss of motor skills, worsening mood, and addiction.

Spinal Cord Stimulation

An electrical stimulator is implanted under the skin, and an electrode is placed next to the spinal cord. The nerve pathways in the spinal cord are stimulated by an electric current. This interferes with the pain impulses traveling toward the brain and lessens the pain felt. Spinal cord stimulation is rooted in what's called the "gate control" theory of pain, which was introduced by Ronald Melzack and Patrick Wall in the 1965 *Science* article "Pain Mechanisms: A New Theory." According to this theory, a metaphorical gate controls the signaling of pain, and you can give an innocuous stimulus to affect pain fibers and interrupt the flow of pain. This helps explain why, if you rub or shake your hand after you bang your finger, you stimulate a cascade of events that effectively "closes the gate" and reduces the perception of pain. Does this really work? Although there isn't a lot of hard evidence to show how well spinal cord stimulation works, it seems to help those who have failed back syndrome and chronic low back pain. Some researchers have reported that more than half of the people receiving spinal cord stimulation for chronic low back and leg pain, ischemic leg pain (for example, from peripheral arterial disease), or complex regional pain syndrome experienced pain reduction or relief. However, initial pain relief is often followed by a gradual decline in effectiveness, apparently caused by the body's increasing tolerance to the treatment.

Morphine Pump

Morphine pumps ("intrathecal drug delivery") are created to provide very small quantities of medication to the spinal fluid; they are surgically inserted under the skin of your abdomen. A morphine pump contains a metal pump, which stores and delivers the drug, as well as

FOR A LIST of online resources on these strategies, refer to the Recommended Reading and Online Resources section.

a catheter, which delivers it into the spinal fluid so that the medication takes effect. Nowadays there are two variations of this pump. One is a constant pump that delivers the medication at a continual rate, and the other is a programmable pump that delivers the medication according to the specified rate in the program. In general, morphine pumps are a treatment of last resort; they are used once all other traditional methods have failed to relieve long-term symptoms.

Deep-Brain Stimulation

Similar to spinal cord stimulation, an electrical stimulator is placed in the brain using a local anesthetic, and a slight current is delivered that interrupts the pain signal coming into the brain. Some call this device a "pacemaker" for the brain. Because most stimuli end up in the thalamus region of the brain—which is often described as the brain's sensory relay station—stimulating this area affects nerve cell signals that can result in pain. Interestingly, deep-brain stimulation was first developed in France in 1987 and evolved out of the so-called ablative, or lesioning, surgeries in which doctors used heat probes to burn and permanently damage small regions of the brain in hopes of relieving certain symptoms such as those related to Parkinson's disease. Deep-brain stimulation has been shown to be most effective in people with failed back syndrome.

When All Else Fails

If there's one type of patient who gives a wise physician pause, it's the patient who walks into the office declaring any of the following two sets of statements:

- The expectation statements:
  - "Doc, I know that you can cure me."
  - "I hear you're the best!"
- The accusatory statements:
  - "I told 'em the bags were too heavy to lift!"
  - "That floor was wet and I was bound to slip!"

Statements like these also have deep psychological roots—an expectation that can inhibit the healing process for the kinds of pain requiring even the most straightforward treatments.

Patients who express unreasonable expectations or anger and frustration at others (a boss, coworker, family member, and so on) are often so inexorably tied to their strong emotions that they can't give up their fury and allow themselves to heal. They are hurt and resentful, which prevents them from initiating a successful treatment process.

As I've been saying since the first page of this book, one of the best attitudes you can have in seeking optimal care and an ideal outcome is to approach your doctor with a team-oriented perspective. It's well documented that patients are often dissatisfied with treatment for back pain. They feel that their doctors are impatient when it comes to diagnosing and understanding their pain, and may further sense that their doctor is not empathetic enough to the fact that the pain is real.

One important lesson I have learned is that the patients most likely to have success in treating their back pain are those who are open-minded. They choose a physician who is an empathetic listener with expertise in low back pain. They also do their part as a willing patient in the diagnostic and treatment phase.

Remember: Your mind has everything to do with whether or not you'll see a day when back pain doesn't affect your life.

Remember: Regardless of your pain's origin and treatment, it helps to keep realistic expectations with a level of acceptance that you may have to live a highly functioning life with a certain amount of pain. The burgeoning field of pain management is helping chronic low back pain patients deal with discomfort that might have previously led to a lifetime of misery.

And last but not least, always remember this: Pain might be unavoidable, but suffering is always optional.

ACTION PLAN

When your back pain's ground zero is your brain, it can be a challenge to overcome. Below are some questions you need to ask yourself. This will help you determine if your pain needs to be addressed by first looking above your neck. Then you can set a proper course of action.

Tough Questions to Ask Yourself

- Are you addicted to your pain?

If I didn't have pain, my life would be different in the following ways:

*List Three or More **Negative** Consequences to Being Pain-Free:*

1. _____.
2. _____.
3. _____.

*List Three or More **Positive** Consequences to Being Pain-Free:*

1. _____.
2. _____.
3. _____.

- How does your pain serve you? Be honest. List all the ways in which your pain serves you (e.g., you get more attention, you have access to pain medication, you have an excuse to not participate in certain activities or tasks):

  _____

  _____

- Are you seeking care for back pain while you currently deal with other problems at work or in your personal life? If so, how?

  _____

  _____

Step 5

Live a Life That Supports
a Strong, Healthy Back

ARE YOU READING THIS STANDING UP OR SITTING DOWN? IN early 2011, Leah Price wrote a marvelous article in the *New York Times Book Review* called "Bent Spines." In it, she describes her own back pain journey and reviews a history of the "perils" and the dangers of reading. Long before 1949, when the term *ergonomics* joined our vocabulary, doctors blamed reading for all sorts of health hazards, including (to repeat the quote she used from one 1795 authority) "weakening of the eyes, heat rashes, gout, arthritis, hemorrhoids, asthma, apoplexy, pulmonary disease, indigestion, blocking of the bowels, nervous disorder, migraines, epilepsy, hypochondria, and melancholy." Since reading often entails sitting, it can aggravate certain types of back pain. And we know now that prolonged sitting has numerous biological consequences that go beyond just back issues. In the past couple of years, new science has emerged to incriminate extensive sitting in increasing one's overall mortality risk.

It's no surprise then that inventive minds have tried, through the ages, to concoct reading implements to make reading easier and accommodate people who preferred to stand or access multiple books at once. Renaissance inventors designed Ferris wheel–like contraptions in which each volume rides flat on a tray, open to just where the reader left it. Thomas Jefferson imagined a lazy Susan–like bookstand that could hold five books open at once.

Labor- and back-saving devices are probably as old as the libraries in the world. So are devices claiming to be the ultimate back pain remedy. But today we have easier means to market these devices, thanks to the Internet and television.

If you flip on the television late at night or on a Saturday morning, you're likely to encounter infomercials claiming to end your back pain with the purchase of their "revolutionary" device, program, or system. As I write this, I'm fielding questions about one popular device in particular that is currently featured on television with its promise to relieve back pain in a matter of minutes. Do these things work? What do I think of them? It's a straightforward answer: If they work for you, they work for you. At this point in the book, you know that solving back pain problems requires an interdisciplinary approach. And part of that interdisciplinary approach entails trial and error, because there's no way to know exactly why one treatment works miraculously on one patient and does absolutely nothing for another person who seemingly has the same problem. I have no doubt that some of the positive effect of these devices is a result of the placebo effect. But there's nothing wrong with the placebo effect if it eases your pain. As I've been emphasizing throughout this book, pain remains such a mystery to us that it behooves us to try new approaches and be open to options that could have a positive impact. We just also need to be careful about making too many assumptions and throwing all of our faith (and money) into products that claim to generate miraculous results. So, should you try something that shouts out to you on late-night television? That's up to you. It's unlikely that it will hurt (except for your wallet), and it just might help.

Aside from these devices marketed to you (often by people with no medical or doctoral degrees), there are a variety of other "treatments" that actually don't require much money, if any, at all. This chapter is going to guide you through the most accessible—and effective—ways in which you can reap the benefits of these options that are really, more than anything, simply elements of a healthy lifestyle. They are the most influential factors in maintaining a lifelong strong and healthy back, and they encompass the following:

- Maintaining good posture.
- Staying mobile and active.
- Savoring sound sleep.

- Adopting a positive attitude.
- Eating well.

I will discuss each of these thematic prescriptions separately, but as a whole they constitute a marvelous recipe for giving yourself an advantage in managing, treating, and preventing back pain. Some of these ideas have already been mentioned in earlier parts of this book, but here I'm going to focus squarely on how you can incorporate each of these key aspects of a pain-free life into your own daily living.

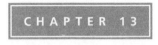

CHAPTER 13

Harness the Power of Posture, Movement, Sleep, Positive Thinking, and a Healthy Diet

F YOU WANT TO GET a good look at a healthy spine, just look at a toddler sitting on the floor. Think of her perfect posture and how easily she moves from one position to another. Now look at yourself. What has happened that has diminished your range of motion? How do you maintain the biomechanical advantage of a three-year-old? Does your spine allow you to move through enough range of motion to engage in normal day-to-day activities? Can you turn, bend, and jump? How can you keep your spine healthy? How much is a healthy spine tied to your overall state of well-being? These are just some of the questions you should be asking yourself.

Poor posture is the plague of low back pain. Most of us pay little attention to our posture—how we hold ourselves up and position our bodies when either sitting or standing. As a rule, we slouch, we have poor body mechanics, and we're overweight. Over time, the stress of poor posture may even alter the anatomical characteristics of the spine, and create problems with muscles, discs, and joints. Many people could prevent and even be relieved of their low back pain by simply gaining a better awareness of their body's natural mechanics. In fact, good posture bolsters any existing treatment to alleviate low back pain. It's also key to staying young, and as an additional bonus, we look thinner and taller. Posture can actually play a big part in how you look and feel, and can also help you to stay stronger and more flexible as you get older.

Fitness and exercise physiologists focus on posture. They know how important it is in the health equation, and they also know how often people neglect it. When you hunch over or sit with your legs crossed and shoulders slouched over, you can cause compressions that create further imbalance. Certain ligaments get stretched too much while others not enough. You'd be surprised at the extent to which a balanced body (i.e., one with good posture) fosters an enhanced environment for bodily function. Good posture allows the diaphragm to function more efficiently and you breathe more deeply. It decompresses the spine and promotes vertebral alignment. It balances the muscles supporting the spine and creates what I like to call a sense of "ease"—ease that facilitates joints so that they function effortlessly and without pain.

I think everyone can improve his or her posture. Here are some basic tips to working on your posture:

• First, try to correct your slouching habits on your own. Stand up and lift your chin slightly; align your ears over your shoulders and your shoulders over your hips. Place your hands on your hips and pitch forward about two inches. There should be a slight inward curve in your lower back, an outward curve in your upper back, and another inward curve at your neck. Maintain this posture and sit down.

- When you are sitting or driving for long periods of time, place a cushion or rolled-up towel between the curve of your lower spine and the back of your seat. By supporting your lower back, you will maintain the natural curve of your spine; when the back is supported, the shoulders fall more naturally into place.

- Maintaining good posture requires abdominal and back strength. Consider classes that focus on core strength, such as yoga or Pilates, as well as stretching. Developing your core—the muscles and connective tissues that hold the spine in place—will automatically help you to maintain proper posture, and stretching helps break bad patterns and allows your muscles to return to neutral. Or hire a physical therapist to create a personalized exercise plan (more on this later).

- Attention, cubicle dwellers: If you sit at a desk all day, see if you can pull your chest up (avoid slouching forward or leaning back), with shoulders down (not up by your ears) and relaxed with your head lined up right over them. If you find yourself sitting for long periods of time, make it a habit of checking in with yourself every twenty minutes or so to make sure you haven't gotten lazy in your posture. If you have a desk job, invest in an ergonomic chair. Ask your human resources department if they have an ergonomics expert on staff (some large companies do) who can assess your work area. An ergonomist can make sure your chair, desk, and keyboard are at the optimal height and can adjust your sitting posture. If no expert is on hand, make adjustments yourself. The center of your computer screen should be at eye level, and the desk height should allow your forearms to rest comfortably at a ninety-degree angle. Work with your feet flat on the floor and your back against the chair.

- Avoid sitting for long lengths of time, which puts pressure on discs and fatigues muscles. Whether you work in an office or at home, get up and stretch every thirty to sixty minutes. Most workers spend the majority of their days—upwards of 8.5 hours on average—sitting down. Try the following at intervals throughout the day: Stand up and place your hands on your lower back, as if you were sliding them into your back pockets. Gently push your hips forward and slightly arch your back. Sit back down and circle your shoulders backward, with your chin tucked, about ten times.

- Can't remember to call a back time-out? How many of us find ourselves slouched over a keyboard after we've logged on to the Internet long ago? Set your phone or computer alarm to remind you to stand up and stretch each hour. An iPhone app called Alarmed has a feature that allows you to create regular reminders throughout the day.

Here's a challenge: See if you can go a day without cradling a cell phone in between your ear and shoulder; switch which shoulder carries the purse, and rely on the hand that doesn't normally carry items to lift and tote. Taking up yoga, Pilates, the Alexander Technique, or the Feldenkrais Method can also help you focus on posture; these practices are all about finding body balance and strengthening the muscles that will naturally allow you to maintain good posture.

Ending Back Pain Through Exercise

It sounds counterintuitive. How can movement, especially movement that works the spine, improve back pain rather than exacerbate it? It's no secret that exercise does a body good, and I know that I'm not the first person to tell you about its benefits. But what about exercise on a bad back? The research is well documented: Exercise does a bad back good. For most people with low back pain, physical activity plays a strong role in recovery from back pain and especially in helping prevent future pain and loss of function. A recent study found that exercising four days a week gave people greater relief from back pain than those who worked out fewer times per week or not at all. Two other studies in particular that reviewed massive amounts of data prove the power of exercise in addressing back pain. In 2004, Sarah D. Liddle and colleagues from Northern Ireland performed a systematic review of randomized controlled trials on exercise for chronic and recurrent low back pain. They asked a simple question: What works? Their studies consisted of any array of patients, from those with simple back pain to individuals who had filed workers' compensation claims. The most common form of exercise used in many of the studies was supervised strength training and, in some cases, flexibility exercises. The results were clear: All sixteen trials demonstrated that chronic low back pain patients achieve positive results following exercise therapy.

In a second study, Dr. James Rainville and his associates from Boston looked at a larger body of evidence from both observational and controlled trials. His results also confirmed the value in exercise, concluding that exercise could improve back-related function, reduce pain and disability, and lead to improvements in pain-related fears, anxieties, and activity-avoidant behavior.

Because exercise has been shown to have such wide-reaching effects on the body, from fighting the onset of age-related disease to boosting your mood and sense of well-being, it makes sense that a lack of exercise has been linked to several chronic diseases, including chronic back pain. In the past, few physicians asked their patients about their exercise habits, but thankfully that is changing. There's a growing movement spearheaded by the American College of Sports Medicine to have physicians and other health care providers query their patients about their exercise habits at every general medical consultation. We're typically asked about smoking and drinking habits, but not always about our physical activity habits. I suspect that this is because most physicians are not trained in the benefits of exercise and they are uncertain their patients will be receptive to exercise advice. This is especially true if the physicians themselves don't look like they should be playing the part of dispensing such advice!

That all said, you should be mindful that the wrong kind of exer-

THE BENEFITS OF exercise have long been reported and proven. All of the following benefits circle back to have a positive influence on your body and ability to maintain your youthful back:

- Increased stamina and energy.
- Increased flexibility.
- Increased blood circulation and enhanced cardiovascular system.
- Increased lung capacity and oxygen supply to cells and tissues.
- More restful, sound sleep.
- Reduction in stress.
- Increased self-esteem and improved mood, and sense of well-being.
- Increased muscle strength, tone, and endurance.
- Release of brain chemicals called endorphins that act as natural tranquilizers.
- Decreased blood sugar levels and risk for diabetes.
- Decreased inflammation.
- Weight distribution and maintenance.

cise, or the correct exercise done incorrectly, can do a lot of damage or exacerbate an existing condition. For instance, I have many patients who love to run. Unfortunately, running doesn't always love them or their backs.

On the following pages, I'm going to outline some of the exercises that I recommend to my patients. A key point to remember is that all exercise programs should be individualized because people have distinct levels of pain and differing injuries that caused the pain initially. Above all, it's important to strengthen the core and back muscles—this should be the essential goal of any exercise program for low back pain. A doctor, physical therapist, or physiatrist is usually the best equipped to help you tailor an appropriate exercise program to meet your individual needs.

The Workout

Just as reinforced steel can bear more weight than sheet aluminum, a strong, well-conditioned back can withstand more stress, and protect the spine better, than a back that has not been conditioned through exercise. Ideally, a well-rounded and comprehensive exercise program includes cardio work, as well as strength training and flexibility exercises. These activities afford you the unique benefits your body needs to achieve peak performance and maintain any pain management program. All of them, collectively, will keep your body moving and also help you maintain good posture. The type of activity you do is not nearly as important as how often you do it and how long you do it. It's important to keep a regular, daily routine rather than save up your tickets to exercise for the weekend. Otherwise, you could very well damage your back more by suddenly forcing it to do things it's not prepared for.

If you've been sedentary or you've avoided exercise for fear that it will hurt your back more, then of course you'll have to ease your way back into a routine.

What about sciatica patients? While it may seem counterintuitive here, too, activity is usually better for relieving sciatic pain than bed rest. Patients may rest for a day or two after their sciatic pain flares

A PHYSICAL THERAPIST, chiropractor, physiatrist (PM and R, or physical medicine and rehabilitation physician), certified athletic trainer (ATC), or other spine specialist who treats the leg pain and other symptoms associated with sciatica will typically prescribe specific exercises and teach the patient how to do those exercises.

up, but after that time period, inactivity will usually make the pain worse. Without exercise and movement, the back muscles and spinal structures become deconditioned and less able to support the back. The deconditioning and weakening can lead to back strain, which causes additional pain.

Get Back into Shape

It's never too late to get back into shape, even if you've been through hell and back with your pain—and even if you still hesitate about the thought of exercise. First, have a conversation with your doctor or, in some cases, with a physical therapist about your unique circumstances. Depending on your age and any chronic diseases and conditions, you may need to consider certain limitations or recommendations that keep you safe and injury-free. Then heed the following tips:

- *Make movement a part of daily life.* Consciously think about moving more throughout your daily routines—literally. Take the stairs instead of the elevator, walk instead of drive to your local market to pick up an item. Find ways to be more active naturally.
- *Pace yourself.* Don't attack a new exercise program like an Olympic athlete. Go slowly and set realistic goals for you and your body. Your cardiovascular, musculoskeletal, and respiratory systems are three big networks in your body that will need to adapt to your new routine, so be patient. Start with short, ten-minute intervals of low-impact activity, which can be as simple as walking. Or try a stationary bike or elliptical machine. Stay at a pace that allows you to maintain a conversation without feeling breathless. Gradually increase the frequency and duration of your daily exercise. Aim to build your program up until you can do thirty to sixty minutes at least five days a week.
- *Give yourself permission to feel "pain".* No one starts a new exercise

program without some pain, even if it's just the pain of spent muscles, feeling more tired, or feeling like you're winded. Your body will adjust over time, but it will go through a "breaking in" period during which you may not feel all the amazing benefits that people talk about when it comes to exercise. I like to remind my patients that there's a difference between hurt and harm. Some exercise may cause you some hurt, but it's unlikely to actually harm you.

- *Build a baseline with weights.* To help make aerobic exercise easier, it helps to also build stronger muscles through strength training. This can be done twice a week with weights, exercise machines, or stretch bands. Just don't do these exercises on consecutive days, as your muscles will need time to recover. The personal trainer at your gym can help you design a comprehensive program that targets all the muscle groups.

- *Dress and drink the part.* Obviously, you won't work out in jeans or high heels. Wear loose clothing and comfortable, supportive shoes. In fact, your shoe preference should be selective even when you're not working out: Ease the strain on your knees, back, and feet by wearing highly supportive shoes. Stay hydrated by drinking eight glasses of water each day, and more when you work out.

- *Seek a support system.* It helps to have at least one exercise buddy with whom you can share walks and exercise classes, and who can encourage you to try new challenges. Being accountable to someone will also compel you to schedule exercise into your life no matter what.

Do Your Cardio

Sometimes called simply "aerobics," this form of exercise gets your heart rate up for an extended period of time, which tones your cardiovascular system. Aerobic exercise increases the flow of blood and nutrients to the back, which supports healing, and can decrease the stiffness in the back and joints that lead to back pain. While many patients with back pain are able to participate in vigorous exercise, such as running or step aerobics, others find it easier to engage in low-impact exercise, such as swimming or cycling, which does not jar the spine.

Patients who regularly undertake aerobic exercise to condition the back will benefit in several ways: (1) They have fewer episodes of low back pain, and will experience less pain when an episode occurs; (2) they are more likely to stay functional—continuing to work and carrying on with recreational activities; (3) they find it easier to control weight or lose weight, decreasing the stress placed on the spine structures and joints; and (4) they experience the biochemical effects of exercise that trigger the release of natural pain-relieving chemicals in their bodies, many of which can elevate mood and relieve symptoms of depression, which you know by now is a common condition in back pain sufferers.

I highly advise that you start with low-impact exercises if you're not already participating in higher-impact activities without any issues to your back. There are several types of cardio exercises that are gentle on the back and, when done on a regular basis, highly effective in providing conditioning. Whatever low-impact exercise is used, the exercise should be vigorous enough to increase the heart rate to the target zone (which is scaled to the age of the patient) and keep it elevated. Elevating the heart rate for at least twenty minutes is required to improve cardiovascular strength, burn excess calories, and make noticeable strides in fitness.

Some ideas:

Walking. It doesn't get any easier than this exercise, both in terms of access and equipment. All you need is a good pair of shoes suitable for walking. Aim to walk most days of the week for a couple of miles at a time. Gradually increase your mileage or the intensity of your walks with hills. It can be done inside or outside, in almost any location, including at home on a treadmill.

Stationary bicycling. For those patients who are more comfortable seated rather than standing, biking or stationary biking may be preferable. Bicycling or "spinning" classes have grown in popularity over the last decade as more people realize the benefits of this lower-impact form of exercise. There are several upright and recumbent (reclining) bikes that can be purchased for home use, and many come with programs preloaded so that patients have a good variety of sessions from which to choose.

Elliptical trainer or step machine. These machines provide a low-impact workout because the participant is using pedals suspended above the ground to move in a continuous oval motion, as opposed to continuously stepping on a hard surface. The motor on the machine facilitates a smoother step or forward glide motion, which is less jarring than walking. The benefit of these machines is that they provide an aerobic workout as well as some strengthening or resistance training. Most cross-training machines allow you to engage your arms as well, thus working the upper body. The combination of motions between your feet and arms makes for greater muscle exertion to maintain the movement.

Hydrotherapy. Doing exercises in the water provides for effective conditioning while minimizing stress on the back because the buoyancy of water counteracts the gravitational pull that can compress the spine. When "unweighted" in water, a person becomes more mobile, and stretching and strengthening exercises are less painful. For most people, exercises such as hip abduction lifts, bicep curls, arm circles to exercise deltoids and shoulders, and triceps kickbacks are all easier done in water. All these muscles build strength in the low back or neck, and reduce back pain. Aqua therapy exercise is especially useful for patients in too much pain to tolerate land exercises on a mat or hard floor, or for elderly patients.

Do Strength Training and Flexibility Work

Technically, strength training employs the use of weights or elastic bands, or in some cases even your own body weight, as resistance. It will keep your bones strong and prevent the loss of lean muscle mass that naturally occurs with age. And it will rev your metabolism for an extended period of time so that you can burn more calories—even after your workout is over. There are lots of ways in which you can engage this form of exercise for purposes of strengthening the spinal column in particular as well as the supporting muscles, ligaments and tendons. These exercises can target abdominal (stomach) muscles and gluteus (buttocks) and hip muscles as well. Taken together, these strong "core" muscles can provide back pain relief because they provide strong support for the spine, keeping it in alignment and facilitating movements that extend or twist the spine. Often, the same workouts that strengthen your muscles will also help you become more flexible and less susceptible to joint pain, as many of the strength-training activities also entail stretching.

Two of the most well-known back-strengthening exercises are McKenzie exercises and dynamic lumbar stabilization (described in more detail on page 243). These back exercises are generally first learned by working with a physical therapist who can demonstrate the exercises and correct your form to ensure strengthening and/or back pain relief is achieved. Although McKenzie exercises and dynamic lumbar stabilization exercises tend to be used for specific conditions, the two forms of physical therapy exercise may also be combined when appropriate.

Williams Flexion and McKenzie Extension Exercises

As I discussed earlier, these two sets of exercises have been used for a long time to help treat low back pain. Developed by two physical therapists, based on two different perspectives, each of these separate sets of exercises carries its own potential benefits. Paul Williams preferred the squat and bounce, whereas Robin McKenzie taught patients to extend their spines using a press-up, flex their knees to the chest, or slide sideways—whatever it took to "centralize" their pain. While on the surface these procedures may appear different, keep in mind that each of these clinicians taught their patients to control their back pain through movement.

Dynamic Lumbar Stabilization Exercises

As I noted earlier, a physical therapist performing these exercises on you will first try to find your "neutral" spine, or the position that allows you to feel most comfortable. The back muscles are then exercised to teach the spine how to stay in this position. This back exercise technique relies on proprioception, which, again, is the awareness of where your joints are positioned. Performed on an ongoing basis, these back exercises provide pain relief and help keep the back strong and well positioned.

Lumbar stabilization back exercises may also be done in conjunction with McKenzie and/or Williams exercises. The McKenzie and Williams exercises serve to reduce back pain, and the lumbar stabilization exercises help strengthen the back. Stabilization back exercises can be rather rigorous and therefore may not be well tolerated by all patients. It may be advisable for elderly patients or patients in significant pain to use other, less strenuous means of physical therapy and exercise to strengthen the back.

The important aspect is that the exercise includes controlled, pro-

TYPICAL MCKENZIE BACK EXTENSION EXERCISES

(Source: Backtrainer.com)

1. **PRONE LYING.** Lie on your stomach with your arms along your sides and head turned to one side. Maintain this position for five to ten minutes.

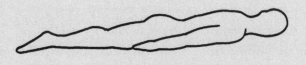

2. **PRONE LYING ON ELBOWS.** Lie on your stomach with your weight on your elbows and forearms and your hips touching the floor or mat. Relax your lower back. Remain in this position for five to ten minutes. If this causes pain, repeat exercise 1, then try again.

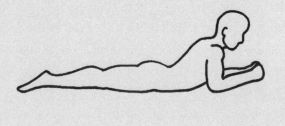

3. **PRONE PRESS-UPS.** Lie on your stomach with your palms near your shoulders, as if to do a standard push-up. Slowly push your shoulders up, keeping your hips on the surface and letting your back and stomach sag. Slowly lower your shoulders. Repeat ten times.

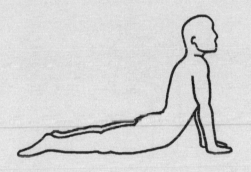

4. **PROGRESSIVE EXTENSION WITH PILLOWS.** Lie on your stomach and place a pillow under your chest. After several minutes, add a second pillow. If this does not hurt, after a few more minutes add a third pillow. Stay in this position for up to ten minutes. Remove pillows one at a time over several minutes.

5. **STANDING EXTENSION.** While standing, place your hands in the small of your back and lean backward. Hold for twenty seconds and repeat. Use this exercise after normal activities during the day that place your back in a flexed position (lifting, forward bending, sitting, etc.)

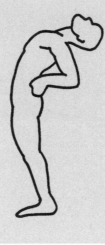

EXAMPLES OF WILLIAMS FLEXION EXERCISES
(Source: Wikipedia.com)

1. **PELVIC TILT.** Lie on your back with your knees bent and your feet flat on the floor. Flatten the small of your back against the floor, without pushing down with your legs. Hold for five to ten seconds.

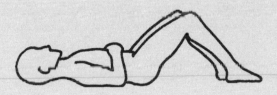

2. **SINGLE KNEE TO CHEST.** Lie on your back with your knees bent and your feet flat on the floor. Slowly pull your right knee toward your shoulder and hold for five to ten seconds. Lower your right knee and repeat with your left knee.

3. **DOUBLE KNEE TO CHEST.** Begin as in the previous exercise. After pulling your right knee to your chest, pull your left knee to your chest and hold both knees for five to ten seconds. Slowly lower one leg at a time.

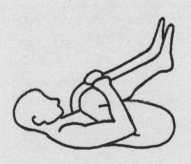

4. PARTIAL SIT-UP. Do the pelvic tilt first and, while holding this position, slowly curl your head and shoulders off the floor. Hold briefly. Return slowly to the starting position.

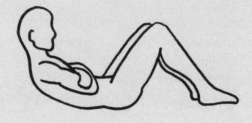

5. HAMSTRING STRETCH. Start in a long sitting position with your toes directed toward the ceiling and your knees fully extended. Slowly lower your trunk forward over your legs, keeping your knees extended, arms outstretched over your legs, and eyes focused ahead.

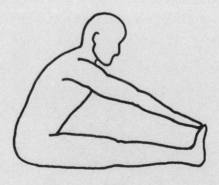

6. **HIP FLEXOR STRETCH.** Place one foot in front of the other with your left (front) knee flexed and your right (back) knee held rigidly straight. Flex forward through your trunk until your left knee contacts the axillary fold (armpit region). Repeat with your right leg forward and left leg back.

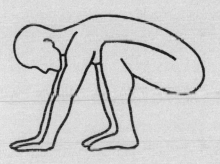

7. **SQUAT.** Stand with both feet parallel, about shoulder-width apart. While attempting to maintain your trunk as perpendicular as possible to the floor, with your eyes focused ahead and feet flat on the floor, slowly lower your body by flexing your knees.

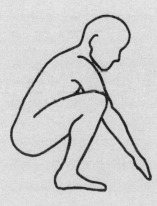

gressive strengthening exercises. Alternative forms of strengthening exercise that can be gentle on the back include Pilates, yoga, and tai chi. There are several forms of these disciplines, and they are best learned working with a certified trainer or practitioner.

Bear in mind that while moderate exercise has profound anti-inflammatory and antistress effects, heavy and prolonged exercise releases huge quantities of stress hormones, so the key is to find a balance. Listen to your body. Listen to your back.

Sleeping off Back Pain

We know so much more now about the effects of sleep on the body from both a psychological and physical standpoint. Pain and poor sleep tend to travel in vicious cycles: Pain makes restful sleep difficult, and a restless night of sleep makes managing the pain all the more challenging. An estimated 50 to 70 percent of pain patients don't get the quality sleep they need because their pain interferes with a good night's sleep. Americans get nearly an hour less sleep a day than they did forty years ago. Juggling work and family life seems to be the primary sleep robber. No doubt chronic pain is another big thief in the bedroom.

What your body does from the time it slips into bed until the time it wakes you up might have more to do with your pain experience than you realize. New findings in sleep medicine are currently revolutionizing how we think about the value sleep brings to our lives. Cutting-edge science now shows how critical sleep is to our ability to stay focused, learn new things and remember old things, lose fat and keep excess weight off, maintain our moods and sense of well-being, and generally lower the risks for a slew of health problems, such as heart disease, obesity, cerebrovascular disease, and even chronic pain. Sleep can dictate whether you can fight off infections, stave off depression, and how well you can cope with stress. And that's just the tip of the proverbial iceberg when it comes to associations between sleep and well-being.

Contrary to what you might think, sleep is a state of high activity. Seemingly magical events happen when you're sleeping that just cannot take place when you're awake, and which help keep you healthy, strong, and pain-free. For starters, lots of hormones are associated with sleep, some of which rely on shuteye to work. As soon as you enter deep sleep, about twenty to thirty minutes after you first close your eyes, your pituitary gland at the base of your brain begins to pump out high levels of growth hormone (GH)—the most it's going to secrete in twenty-four hours. Not only does growth hormone stimulate growth and cell reproduction, but it renews almost every cell in the body, including those in your bones, vertebrae, and vital organs. It also supports the immune system, and even helps prevent osteoporosis. Without adequate sleep, GH can't circulate from the pituitary.

So, what does an insomniac with back pain do to achieve more restful sleep? I realize that there's no magic bullet to solving all sleep troubles quickly. Neither over-the-counter sleep aids nor serious prescription medications can permanently rescue the poor sleeper. However, just being aware of the role of sleep in your pain experience can give you the motivation you need to focus on creating healthy sleep habits, or what some call healthy "sleep hygiene." Below are some tips, courtesy of Dr. Michael Breus, from his 2007 book *Beauty Sleep*:

Get on a schedule. Go to bed and wake up at the same time seven days a week, weekends included. Try not to fall into a cycle of burning the midnight oil on Sunday night in preparation for Monday, letting your sleep debt pile up for the week and then attempting to catch up on sleep over the weekend. It won't work. Your body and back will love it if you stick to a consistent sleep schedule every day.

Back away from the stimulants early enough. Caf-feinated drinks should be reduced, if not banished, early in the afternoon (at least four to six hours before bedtime). Set aside at least thirty minutes before bedtime to unwind and prepare for sleep. Avoid stimulating activities (e.g., work, being on the computer, watching TV dramas that get your adrenaline run-ning). Once you're in bed, do some light reading and push any anxieties aside.

Try some aromatherapy. Keep a sachet of lavender by your bed and take a whiff before hitting the pillow. Lavender has known sleep-inducing effects. Other aromas widely con-sidered to be relaxing are rose, vanilla, and lemongrass—but different ones work for different people. Experiment. Scented lotions can also be effective.

Can't sleep within twenty to thirty minutes? Then get out of the bedroom. Lying restless in bed, hoping sleep will come quickly, can do more harm than good. The longer we wait, the faster our minds tend to run, triggering more restless, stimulating stress. If you can't get to sleep within a reasonable time period, say twenty to thirty minutes, get out of bed and go to a comfortable place that has dim lighting and no distractions. Just sit comfortably and read or do some breathing exercises. The point is to give your mind a respite from trying so hard to nod off. After twenty minutes or so, go back to bed and see what happens when you're more relaxed. Repeat once or twice if necessary.

Earlier I described the role of emotions in the pain experience. Well, consider the following: Have you ever noticed that the day after a sleepless night you're more emotional, often overreacting to things that you normally would shrug off? We're beginning to figure out why, thanks to some University of California–Berkeley, researchers who kept a group of healthy men and women awake for up to thirty-five hours straight, and then monitored their brains while they showed them a series of pictures that ranged from neutral to aversive. At the sight of the unpleasant photos, their sleep-deprived brains lit up like a firestorm in an area of the brain—the amygdala—that is an emotional center, alerts the body during danger, and activates the fight-or-flight response.

Normally, other parts of the brain weigh in and release chemicals that calm the amygdala. But when you are functioning on zero sleep, things go haywire: The amygdala stays in overdrive, which keeps the stress response going in an endless feedback loop. Bottom line: Sleep helps keep our emotions on an even keel. So, do what you can to achieve restful sleep on a regular basis to give your back a break.

Can You *Think* Your Way out of a Bad Back?

It's a provocative idea, and one that surely has plenty of anecdotal evidence to support it. I just discussed the fact that sleep deprivation throws your emotional center of gravity out of whack, so imagine what that can mean for thoughts on pain—the *perception* of pain—and your motivation for having optimistic feelings about the future of your pain. As with sleep medicine, the field of positive psychology has grown immensely in the last decade or so, and we now have a much greater understanding about the science of stress, how certain psychological stress can affect physiology, and how combating stress with positivity can actually reverse the domino effects that take place in the body to perpetuate illness and even chronic pain.

The scientific study of the impact of stress on the body has also made tremendous advances in the past two decades. In 1998, doctors from Harvard University led a study to understand the interactions between the mind and the body. They dubbed their findings the NICE network, which stands for neuro-immuno-cutaneous-endocrine. Put simply, it's an interconnected network consisting of your nervous system, immune system, skin, and endocrine (hormonal) system. They communicate via certain biochemicals.

The researchers examined how various forces impact our state of mind, from massage and aromatherapy to depression and isolation. What they discovered confirmed what we've already known anecdotally for centuries: Our mental state has a definite influence on our health and even our appearance. People suffering from depression, for example, look older and less healthy than their happier counterparts of the same age. The stress of living with depression has accelerated the aging process and damaged their health. Surely the same conclusion can be made for people living with chronic pain, such as back pain.

The idea that we can proactively change the course of our body's health just through positive thoughts comes at a good time: We live in a world that increasingly makes us feel time deprived, anxious, overworked, and stressed out, all of which, as I just stated, put tremendous pressure on our biological systems. I have no doubt that chronic stress feeds the cycles of chronic pain. Acute and episodic stress, such as the stress that accompanies public speaking or trying to get to work on time every day, aren't nearly as damaging as chronic stress. Chronic stress is the worst kind and can be debilitating. This is the stress that people feel when they cannot see a way out of a miserable situation, and there are plenty of examples here: an unhappy marriage, an ongoing struggle with your (teenage) kids, a serious health challenge, financial troubles, a horrible job, or no job at all. The economic events of the past few years have led to an epidemic of chronic stress in our world. Those who experience chronic stress tend to lack good coping skills, so they ruminate on regrets and worry about the future. They can't find optimism amid all the pessimism.

Try Journaling

Adopting a positive attitude is easier said than done, but I can attest to the power of this approach just from watching my own patients. There are those patients who generally have a sunnier demeanor than others, who don't carry a wet blanket around, and who seem to weather the storm of their back pain a lot better. Their outcomes are also better, as they typically have much higher rates of recovery from chronic pain. Remember, the brain is wired for pain, but it's also wired for pleasure, which can have a direct impact on those pain signals by releasing natural pain-relieving chemicals.

So, no matter where you are in your own emotional journey, it helps to examine your attitude and perspectives. Do you see the glass as half-empty or half-full? Earlier in the book, I asked you to consider the yellow flags that correlate unceasing pain with deeply rooted emotional underpinnings. Now I'm going to ask you to revisit your inventory of potential yellow flags, and challenge you to begin making those emotional shifts that can help you treat and manage your pain for life. How can this be done?

You'd be surprised by what taking just three to five minutes at the start or end of your day to evaluate how you feel and what you're thinking can do for your sense of well-being, peace of mind, and even your capacity to heal your own pain and realize optimal wellness. Indeed, committing your thoughts and ideas to paper can also make a huge difference. It affords you a record from which to look back in the future and simultaneously offers accountability. It also gives you a chance to adjust your attitudes if need be and set a new course that moves you closer to where you want to be. Find a comfortable spot (or just do this exercise while sitting in bed) and consider playing some relaxing music.

I frequently ask my patients to think about the following four questions. Even if you don't choose to write out your responses, think about these questions and take a few minutes to reflect on your answers:

1. How would your world change if you didn't have any issues with your back? In other words, what would you do if you were absolutely pain-free today?
2. What job or hobby would you like to try, especially one that you've avoided because of your pain?
3. Aside from healing your pain, what's the one thing you hope to accomplish in your lifetime that you haven't yet?
4. Aside from your back pain, what in life is causing you a great deal of stress and anxiety? How can you begin to remedy that one step at a time?

You may find it helpful to divide your journal into sections. One section can be designated for writing down the more mundane tasks you need to get gone, such as picking up clothes from the cleaner's, grocery shopping, or organizing a birthday party. Another section can keep track of your diet choices and physical activities. Yet another section can be reserved for recording your personal thoughts and ideas, from troublesome worries to positive notes on the good things you've accomplished. Sometimes you'll find that the act of writing down a worry will lead to solutions that you never thought of before. And, likewise, keeping a written record of your achievements and the experiences that bring you joy can help you to buffer the negative and its physical consequences. All of these exercises will subconsciously give you hope for your future. This exercise may even inspire you to turn a negative into a positive just by reshaping your attitude.

Manage Stress Better

In addition to being reflective routinely, it also helps to have a plan for managing the stress in your life. Stress will always be part of our lives—and our livelihoods. The key is to keep certain sources of un-necessary stress at bay so they don't affect us like a charging bull. Again, easier said than done, but here are some things to consider:

Try something new. Take a class in a subject area you know nothing about. Find a new hobby. Choose to do something you've never done before. It will challenge you in fresh ways, and inspire you to have a more positive outlook on life. Engaging in fun, novel activities can be surprisingly fulfilling and relaxing. Happiness has gained a lot of at-tention in recent years, as volumes of books and studies have emerged to help explain what makes us happy, or not. One of the prevailing pieces of wisdom from the studies on happiness defines it as the pur-suit of engaging and meaningful activities. And there's nothing more engrossing than trying something new that you might come to love.

Don't lose your friends over your pain. Researchers are only now starting to pay attention to the importance of friendship and social networks in overall health. Managing chronic pain can often leave one isolated and avoiding social situations. The pain takes over any semblance of nor-malcy in life. If your pain has changed how you interact with others and maintain friendships, see what you can do to change that. See if you can plan more time with the people who inspire and de-stress you. Regular quality time with the people dear to us can be incredibly ther-apeutic. Strengthening those connections in real life can be as power-ful as any other strategy to boost health and well-being. Research from around the world shows that keeping trusty circles of friends promotes health and longevity. In 2008, Harvard researchers in particular re-ported that strong social ties could promote brain health as we age. Brain health, as I've shown, could be key to staving off pain.

Have more touching moments. The healing power of touch is grossly underestimated in our society, yet it can be one of the most potent tools in health care. Massage not only benefits the muscles and tissues being kneaded and stretched but it also has been found to lower stress levels significantly. It's been shown to increase weight gain in premature infants, alleviate depression, reduce pain in cancer patients, improve sleep patterns, and positively alter the immune system—all of which spell a recipe for pain relief. A class of nerve fibers in the skin called the C-tactile nerve fibers appear to be responsible for sending feel-good messages to the brain upon stimulation through pleasurable touch. Healing-touch therapy can take many forms, not just classic massage. Experiment with different forms of massage that take into consideration your particular back issues.

Practice slow, controlled breathing. As noted earlier, this is the foundation for many Eastern practices, such as yoga, chi gong, tai chi, and classic meditation—all of which aim to immerse the body (and mind, clearly) into a balanced, stress-free state. One of the reasons why deep breathing is so helpful is that it triggers a parasympathetic nerve response, as opposed to a sympathetic nerve response, the latter of which is sensitive to stress and anxiety. At the onset of stress, the sympathetic nervous system springs into action and is largely responsible for those often damaging spikes in the stress hormones cortisol and adrenaline. The parasympathetic nervous system, on the other hand, can trigger a relaxation response, and deep breathing is the quickest means of getting these two systems to communicate. You can flip the switch from high alert to low in seconds as your heart rate slows, muscles relax, and blood pressure lowers.

Deep breathing can be done anywhere, anytime. Sit comfortably in a chair or lie down. Close your eyes and make sure your body is relaxed, releasing all tension in your neck, arms, legs, and back. Inhale through your nose for as long as you can, feeling your diaphragm and abdomen rise as your stomach moves outward. Sip in a little more air when you think you've reached the top of your lungs. Slowly exhale to a count of twenty, pushing every breath of air from your lungs. Continue for at least five rounds of deep breaths.

Stop catastrophizing, or try cognitive behavior therapy. The sky is *not* falling. Having a doomsday attitude about your life and health is one of the classic yellow flags. It's very easy for the mind to exaggerate and distort the magnitude and significance of bad things that happen, and the speed with which you need to remedy them. Just think of the last time you let your thoughts about your back pain morph into thinking (and perhaps believing) that life as you knew it was about to end and that you'd never get back to pain-free living. Anxieties can quickly turn relatively harmless negative circumstances into utter catastrophes.

For this very reason, cognitive behavior therapy (CBT) is very useful in pain management. As its name implies, CBT is partly cognitive and partly behavioral. The cognitive portion is about identifying, challenging, and changing the ways of thinking that leave you stressed. When your mind is awash in negative thoughts, you're likely exaggerating or distorting those thoughts to the extent that they create undue stress. In other words, you're giving your worries too much attention. If you could replace them with positive thoughts related to the problem, however, you can eviscerate the worry.

Countering negative thoughts with a positive one related to the problem takes practice. If you can't hire a CBT therapist who is trained in teaching you how to do this, you can at least start by keeping a journal that records the good things that happen. The exercise can shift the focus to what you're doing right, and that can put a brake on the stressful, negative mental "chatter" that often goes on in our heads. Deep breathing and meditative exercise can also help you.

Dietary Approaches

Clearly, you already know in your heart that taking care of yourself sets the tone of your life and health. I've just covered the four areas in one's lifestyle that can certainly have an influence, however big or small, in one's personal story of pain. If you can sit, stand, exercise, sleep, and think your way to a better back, then what about eating? How much can food play into the pain equation? Can you eat your way out of back pain?

This area of study is probably the least understood, but it bears some consideration.

Can Food Be Your Pain Medicine?

Food has long been a source of healing in medicine, with the exception of one particular field: back pain. For reasons that are not clear, back pain researchers have been reluctant to consider the possibility that foods might have curative properties for sufferers. That reluctance is slowly changing as evidence has begun to build, showing benefits to foods' constituent compounds, which may relieve pain, decrease inflammation, and serve as antioxidants. Granted, you're not going to find any wonder pain relievers in food aisles of your local supermarket, but there's something to be said for incorporating certain foods into your daily regimen that may add to your therapeutic arsenal. So, which foods could potentially alleviate pain? The research is still in its infancy, but so far there's some good news coming from studies of soybean oil, sucrose, and brightly colored fruits and vegetables, which are chock-full of compounds with antioxidant and anti-inflammatory effects. Tart cherries in particular have been known to relieve pain associated with arthritis and gout. Can they address a bad back? The jury is still out, but if you like cherries, then I won't dissuade you from trying. Nutritional medicine is a rapidly expanding subject area today, and we'll no doubt come to learn more about which foods can have potent yet natural anti-pain effects in the body. I've always believed that a healthy diet goes a long way toward maintaining a healthy, pain-free body. Although the halls of research have only begun to reveal clues to how diet influences pain processes, we all would do well to make an effort to improve our diets and consume nutrient-rich foods that may play a role not only in alleviating pain, but also maintaining our overall health.

So-called anti-inflammatory diets have been gaining popularity in recent times. As it becomes increasingly clear that chronic inflammation is the root cause of many serious illnesses, including chronic back pain, people are searching for any way to reduce inflammation, from exercise to diet. I've been using the term *inflammation* a lot throughout this book already, but haven't clearly defined it. We all know inflammation on the surface of the body as local redness, heat, swelling, and pain. It is the cornerstone of the body's healing response, bringing more nourishment and more immune activity to a site of injury or infection. But when inflammation persists or serves no purpose deep inside the body through systemic pathways, it causes illness. Among the many triggers of untamed inflammation are stress, lack of exercise, exposure to toxins such as secondhand smoke, prolonged injury (including a prolonged bout with back pain), and plain old genetic predisposition. Today scientists are learning how diet can also play a role in this process and how certain dietary choices can either fan the flames or, conversely, tame them.

An anti-inflammatory diet is not a diet in the traditional sense— it's not intended as a weight-loss program (although people can and do lose weight on it), nor is it an eating plan to stay on for a limited period of time. Rather, it is way of selecting and preparing foods based on scientific knowledge of how they can help your body maintain optimum health, which entails how the body manages pain. Along with influencing inflammation, such a diet keeps your digestive system healthy and happy, which goes a long way toward promoting feelings of well-being. It also provides steady energy and ample vitamins, minerals, essential fatty acids, dietary fiber, and protective phytonutrients—all of which, again, will support your overall health and wellness.

So, what's in an anti-inflammatory diet? It's pretty simple: Aim to eat a balanced diet filled with colorful whole fruits and vegetables, healthy fats, and lean proteins. Minimize your consumption of processed and fast food, and eat an appropriate amount of calories for your body and activity level. Plenty of other books can show you how to do this meal by meal and snack by snack, so I'm not going to go into those details. For starters, I would recommend checking out Dr. Andrew Weil's site at www.drweil.com, where there is a comprehensive list of anti-inflammatory diet tips to incorporate into your life right away.

Will eating this way relieve back pain? And if so, when? Unfortunately, I cannot answer that. But it's nice to know that with every bite we take, we could be affecting the pro- and anti-inflammatory compounds in the body and tipping the scale in favor of lower inflammation, which in turn could be part of our pain.

I encourage you to experiment with shifts in your diet if you don't already eat healthily and you believe your diet could use a makeover. Even if the benefits of doing so don't directly relieve pain, they can definitely have a positive impact through other benefits that a healthy diet brings. People who eat well tend to have an easier time managing their weight, they don't experience as many issues with digestion and digestive disorders (which tend to present their own forms of pain), and they feel better in general. And it's no secret that when you feel better, you're more apt to do the kinds of things that help manage pain, or heal it entirely.

I've GIVEN YOU a lot of ideas and things to think about in this chapter. I don't expect you to incorporate all of these recommendations into your life today, but try to at least find two actionable steps you can take to at least make one small, doable shift.

ACTION PLAN

- If you don't already engage in the kinds of habits and activities that support a healthy lifestyle, particularly the five key ones outlined in this chapter, then make it a goal to pick one strategy from each of the five and apply it to your life today. Every week, add another strategy.

- See if you can make small chifts in what you've already been doing so that it doesn't seem as if you're making monumental (unrealistic) changes to your life—and that you're not trying to change overnight.

- If you can learn to maintain good posture, stay as active as possible, get a good night's sleep, think optimistically, and eat nutrient-dense foods, then you'll already be on a path to healing, regardless of any other back-specific strategies you employ.

Conclusion:
A Call to Action

FOR THOSE INVOLVED IN the diagnosis, treatment, and management of low back pain, the future has never looked brighter. Many therapies, including those involving stem cells, motion preservation technology, genetic engineering, and surgical techniques, may be the future of low back pain treatment. I hope that we'll continue to decode the mysteries of the bad back and help people tailor personalized treatment protocols to their unique bodies that will ultimately allow them to make the most of their back's mobility—and their lives.

As the subtitle of this book suggests, there are five "steps" to ending back pain using today's technology. But once you started reading, I began to take you on a journey that likely removed you from thinking that you were in fact taking five sequential steps. Why did that happen?

First of all, I wanted to convey to you that treating low back pain lacks the very straightforwardness and one-two-three protocols that so many other areas of medicine enjoy. If you have the flu, you know what to do to treat it. If you break your arm, your doctor will set the bone and immobilize it for a few weeks so that the natural healing process can take place. But in the realm of back pain, not only are the treatments varied and sometimes indirect, but the diagnosis and management of chronic back pain can take a level of effort, patience, time, and tolerance that is just not typical of other health challenges.

My goal in this book has been to show you the complexity of the issues and equip you with at least some knowledge—both basic and clinical—to take control of your back for life.

Now, however, I'm actually going to sum up my main points and recap the five-step road map that you've just learned. All of these should sound familiar. Here they are again in brief:

1. Decipher your back's unique code.
2. Be an advocate for yourself with health professionals.
3. Ensure proper diagnosis.
4. Embark on a plan of treatment and recovery based on your individual diagnosis, one that can entail a wide variety of options from least to most invasive.
5. Take advantage of strategies to prevent future back pain and live as much of a pain-free life as possible.

As a way of summing up these keys and offering a few more reminders, let me end this book with these seven concluding thoughts and recommendations.

Deal with the underlying pain generator. As we've seen, this can involve myriad treatment options, running from the least invasive to surgery if that's appropriate for you. Realize that there may be options, though, that don't include the usual gamut of ideas, such as dietary recommendations to reduce inflammation, meditation, acupuncture, and cognitive therapy that helps you to reduce stress. Remember that the ultimate pain generator can be your brain, and its complex array of deeply seated emotions. Even if you can identify an anatomical pain generator, it still helps to use mind-body therapies to reframe your pain experience and prevent yourself from becoming a chronic pain patient. We all know people who, despite serious struggle and pain in their lives (whether related to their backs or otherwise), live active, joyful, and productive lives. They perceive pain not as the end of the road but as an adversary to be outwitted. They have learned how to think of pain as something in their minds so that it's not cornering them into being victims dependent on others to relieve their suffering. Much to the contrary, they are self-directed individuals who are able to modify their pain and disability through their own thoughts, beliefs, and actions.

Establish a partnership with your doctor. You should feel that you and your doctor are working together as a team, with the goal of arriving at a particular program that helps you manage and treat your back pain, as well as live a normal life. It's been shown that a sense of personal control helps reduce pain and improve the ability to function normally, so it's important for you to take an active role in your treatment and assume responsibility for managing your pain. Likewise, your doctor must make the commitment to take your reports of pain seriously and listen in a caring, respectful way. This in itself can be very healing.

Establish a reliable support system beyond you and your doctor. Managing chronic pain can be incredibly isolating. People who have a strong network of family members and friends tend to weather their pain much better than folks who lack a trusty support system. If you have a significant other (spouse, partner, etc.), or a devoted best friend, try to involve that person in your personal program. Let that person understand your goals, challenges, abilities, and limitations, and when and how to offer support. If you don't have a dependable person or group of people among your friends and family, then don't hesitate to seek such people through pain management programs, your church, and support groups designed for exactly this kind of thing.

Educate yourself. My whole purpose of giving you so many lessons on anatomy, pain, and physiology was to equip you with the knowledge you need to take action and be in control of your pain management.

I've found that patients need to understand what's going on in their bodies before they can begin to manage their health problems. You can learn a lot about what provokes and what diminishes your pain just by keeping a diary, for example. It's one of the best ways to educate yourself about the particularities of your body in addition to the traditional mode of reading and learning about back pain.

A so-called pain diary is a commonly used tool for teasing out pain triggers and determining when and how to best intervene. Doctors keep meticulous records of your pain and track changes when you visit them, but you can keep a much more detailed record yourself and track your pain throughout the day, every day of the week. It couldn't be simpler: Stop several times a day to assess and record the severity (0 to 10 in intensity) and type (sharp, grinding, burning, etc.) of pain that you feel. You can also note what was going on in your day at the time (e.g., sitting at work, moving objects, having an argument with someone), and keep track of what you did to relieve your pain, and whether or not it was effective. Looking back at the end of the week or month, you may be able to see patterns. Maybe the pain gets worse when you're tired or upset, and maybe it improves after you've exercised. Perhaps certain foods trigger pain, and perhaps a stricter diet that's good for your waistline is also good for your pain.

I bet you'll be surprised by what keeping a pain diary can reveal. People are often alarmed at how much they didn't know about their pain before they kept a diary, even though it may have been a familiar and unwelcome companion for a long time. You're likely to pinpoint uncommon triggers of more severe pain, such as certain foods, a sleepless night, stress and anxiety, lack of exercise, and other factors that you can address and change for the better.

Modify behaviors to improve function. One of the most important questions that I ask patients is simply, "What does your pain keep you from doing that you *want* to do?" In other words, back pain aside, which activities are most important to you? The answer to that question helps me design an interdisciplinary program that addresses your needs and your back pain, and set priorities and do whatever is in my power to enable you to continue doing those things and live as "normal" of a life as possible. Again, a pain diary can come in handy here. It can be used to see what triggers your unique discomfort and map out ways to avoid or divert it. Watching your activities to determine how long and how often each can be done without pain helps you learn to pace yourself and set reasonable expectations of what you are able to do. This is where having additional support and guidance can be key. Physical therapists and people who specialize in techniques such as the Alexander Technique or Feldenkrais Method may be able to teach you new ways to perform activities that diminish or help you avoid pain.

Failing to modify your behavior to keep up your body's functioning can have negative effects. I've explained how the behavioral changes that occur once pain sets in can sometimes have unintended consequences. Forgoing exercise, for instance, for fear that it will cause further pain, can often have the reverse effect of worsening the pain and triggering weight gain, which can compound pain. When you hurt, you tend to move about the world differently and change what you do in order to avoid more painful episodes. The other negative result of modifying behavior is that it can provide you a form of excuse. Suddenly, the pain gives you a way out of doing things that you don't want to do. This can be an unconscious choice. You may, for example, find that your pain helps you avoid work that you don't like to perform and taking responsibility for something that you'd rather pass on to someone else. Acknowledging and dealing with these underlying issues can often reduce the severity and frequency of pain.

Increase physical activity. As I described earlier, it may seem counterintuitive to think that exercise, especially the kinds that engage the spine and various back muscles, can reduce back pain, but it's been proven again and again both clinically and anecdotally. Exercise may be the last thing on your mind if you're suffering from debilitating pain, but it has so many benefits that it cannot be ignored. Exercise makes the body just plain feel better, and it does so through a variety of effects—from the release of feel-good endorphins and other biochemicals to its positive effects on muscles, sleep, weight management, self-esteem, sense of empowerment, and overall fitness. Let's not forget that it also eases anxiety, stress, and depression. You may think that exercise will cause more damage, but if you perform the right exercises with the supervision of your doctor and any other therapists who may be helping you in this regard, then chances are good that you'll reduce your pain.

Ease your stress. There are lots of ways in which we can change our perception of pain. It's a foregone conclusion by now: Relieving stress can often work wonders on pain, and especially how we think about pain. While certain kinds of stress, like that experienced on the battlefield, can block pain signals, most kinds of stress we encounter daily do the opposite—they intensify pain sensations. To break the self-perpetuating cycle of tension and pain, it helps to learn and practice regularly a relaxation technique such as meditation, breathing exercises, or progressive muscle relaxation. Or engage in other stress-reducing activities such as physical exercise, yoga, chi gong, a favorite hobby, getting a massage, or visiting a spa, to name a few.

And don't forget the power of positive self-talk. While it may sound corny, telling yourself (even looking in the mirror as you do this), "I won't let the pain stop me. I am in control of this pain and I won't let it control my life" can be very empowering. It's far more helpful than saying, "I can't help myself. I'm doomed. I don't deserve to be healthy and pain-free."

I'M GOING TO END this with a note of congratulations. Just getting this far in the book means you've learned a great deal more about your body and your pain. My hope is that you've achieved a working understanding of the intricacies of your low back pain, and that I've given you plenty of ideas to at least begin to make a tremendous difference in your life. You now appreciate the enormity of this problem and that you're not alone. You also have gained awareness about the back's potential sources of pain and how different pain patterns call for different approaches to alleviate the pain. That awareness alone puts you in a select group of people and will help you to make the changes necessary to live a more pain-free life.

I know the value that being pain-free brings to people because I see it day in, day out. I also see what pain and sickness can do to people, no matter how much success they've experienced in life or how many, and how deeply, people love them. Without a strong and healthy body, you have nothing. But when you do have good health, pretty much anything is possible. Things tend to fall into place when you're healthy and don't have to think about pain. In addition to gaining a more pain-free life, I hope you will also embrace my message's personal call to action. The end of back pain resides within all of us. And it's up to each of us to do what we can to end it.

Whenever possible, keep abreast of the literature and be willing to experiment with new strategies when the research supports their value (remember, visit my website at www.drjackstern.com to access resources). Between the knowledge you've gained in this book and the information that you'll continue to gather as you press forward, you'll be in a position to lobby the medical establishment for the care you need and deserve. Some of you have had to take a long, hard look at yourselves and your relationship with your pain. Some of you may not have liked what you saw. But I'm also hoping that along the way you realized that you can become a functional person once again. This is not only a possibility but a likelihood. Best wishes to you.

Your partner in back health,
Dr. Jack Stern

Acknowledgments

This book could not have been written without the lessons learned from my patients. To them I am eternally grateful.

I am also thankful to my mentors and teachers—some cited in this book, but many more not mentioned—who modeled for me the sacred nature of our profession and the virtue of humility, who instilled in me the passion to cherish human life, and to see the humanity in each person who entrusted me with their care.

To Bonnie Solow, my amazing agent. Since the start, you've stood by this project with an indomitable spirit. It wouldn't have come to fruition without you. Thank you for your patience, vision, leadership, and, above all, friendship. Any author would be lucky to have you in his court.

I am deeply indebted to Kristin Loberg, who transformed my ramblings into accessible, lucid text while still conveying the essence of my message. I am truly fortunate to have found a writing partner who worked so hard combining great intelligence and loving optimism.

Thanks to the incredible team at Avery: Megan Newman, Lisa Johnson, Gigi Campo, Lindsay Gordon, and especially Marisa Vigilante, who beautifully edited the manuscript and helped to turn this giant body of work into a final, polished product.

And to my beloved son, Daniel, who did the illustrations.

I tried as best I could to accurately cite pertinent medical literature, but our knowledge is rapidly changing, so I take full responsibility for any errors or omissions.

Recommended Reading

The following is a partial list of books and scientific papers that you may find helpful in learning more about the ideas and concepts expressed in this book. This is by no means an exhaustive list, but it will get you started in gaining a better understanding of back pain and the current science behind strategies to treat it. These materials can also open other doors for further research and inquiry. For access to more studies and an ongoing updated list of references, please visit www .drjackstern.com. If you do not see a reference listed here that was mentioned in the book, please refer to the website, where a more comprehensive list can be found.

Airaksinen, O, et al. European guidelines for the management of chronic nonspecific low back pain. Chapter 4. *Eur Spine J.* 2006 Mar;15 (Suppl 2):S192–300.

Alyas F, M Turner, and D Connell. MRI findings in the lumbar spines of asymptomatic, adolescent, elite tennis players. *Br J Sports Med.* 2007 Nov;41(11):836-841; discussion 841. Epub 2007 Jul 19.

Baliki, MN, et al. Chronic pain and the emotional brain: specific brain activity associated with spontaneous fluctuations of intensity of chronic back pain. *J Neurosci.* 2006 Nov 22;26(47):1216–12173.

Berkman, L, and AM Epstein. Beyond health care—socioeconomic status and health. *N Engl J Med.* 2008 Jun 5;358(23):2509–2510.

Betz, Sherri R. Modifying pilates for clients with osteoporosis. *IDEA Fitness Journal.* 2005 April. Accessed online at http://www.ideafit .com/fitness-library/pilates-osteoporosis on September 13, 2012.

Bigos, SJ, et al. Back injuries in industry: a retrospective study. II. Injury factors. *Spine* (Phila Pa 1976). 1986 Apr;11(3):246–251.

Bigos, SJ, et al. Back injuries in industry: a retrospective study. III. Employee-related factors. *Spine* (Phila Pa 1976). 1986 Apr;11(3): 252–256.

Bishop, PB, JA Quon, CG Fisher, and MF Dvorak. The Chiropractic Hospital-based Interventions Research Outcomes (CHIRO) study: a randomized controlled trial on the effectiveness of clinical practice guidelines in the medical and chiropractic management of patients with acute mechanical low back pain. *Spine J.* 2010 Dec;10(12):1055–1064.

Björnsdotter, M, I Morrison, and H Olausson. Feeling good: on the role of C fiber mediated touch in interoception. *Exp Brain Res.* 2010 Dec;207(3–4):149–155. Epub 2010 Oct 21.

BMJ Specialty Journals (2007 July 19). Intensive training of young tennis players can cause spinal damage, study shows. *ScienceDaily.* Accessed online at http://www.sciencedaily.com /releases/2007/07 /070719011158.htm on September 11, 2012.

Breus, M. *Beauty Sleep: Look Younger, Lose Weight, and Feel Great.* New York: Plume, 2007.

Buchbinder, R, et al. A randomized trial of vertebroplasty for painful osteoporotic vertebral fractures. *N Engl J Med.* 2009 Aug 6; 361(6):557–568.

Cacciatore, TW, VS Gurfinkel, FB Horak, PJ Cordo, and KE Ames. Increased dynamic regulation of postural tone through Alexander Technique training. *Hum Mov Sci.* 2011 Feb;30(1):74–89. Epub 2010 Dec 23.

Carette, S, et al. A controlled trial of corticosteroid injections into facet joints for chronic low back pain. *N Engl J Med.* 1991 Oct 3;325(14):1002–1007.

Carneiro, KA, and JD Rittenberg. The role of exercise and alternative treatments for low back pain. *Phys Med Rehabil Clin N Am.* 2010 Nov;21(4):777–792.

Carragee, EJ, TF Alamin, JL Miller, and JM Carragee. Discographic, MRI and psychosocial determinants of low back pain disability and remission: a prospective study in subjects with benign persistent back pain. *Spine J.* 2005 Jan–Feb;5(1):24–35.

Chapin, H, E Bagarinao, and S Mackey. Real-time fMRI applied to pain management. *Neurosci Lett.* 2012 Jun 29;520(2):174–181. Epub 2012 Mar 3.

Cherkin, DC, et al. A comparison of the effects of 2 types of massage and usual care on chronic low back pain: a randomized, controlled trial. *Ann Intern Med.* 2011 Jul 5;155(1):1–9.

Cherkin, DC, RA Deyo, M Battié, J Street, and W Barlow. A comparison of physical therapy, chiropractic manipulation, and provision of an educational booklet for the treatment of patients with low back pain. *N Engl J Med.* 1998 Oct 8;339(15):1021–1029.

Chou, R. What are the most important risk factors for chronic disabling low back pain? *The Back Letter.* 2010 Aug;25(8):85,92–93.

Chou, R, and P Shekelle. Will this patient develop persistent disabling low back pain? *JAMA.* 2010 Apr 7;303(13):1295–1302.

deCharms, RC, et al. Control over brain activation and pain learned by using real-time functional MRI. *Proc Natl Acad Sci* USA. 2005 Dec 20;102(51):18626–18631. Epub 2005 Dec 13.

Deyo, R. Rapid growth in spinal injections—without a clear scientific rationale. *The Back Letter.* 2007 Sept;22(9):97,104–105. doi: 10.1097/01.BACK.0000294130.10744.a7.

Deyo, RA, SK Mirza, JA Turner, and BI Martin. Overtreating chronic back pain: time to back off? *J Am Board Fam Med.* 2009 Jan–Feb;22(1):62–68. doi: 10.1097/01.BACK.0000387776.25111.6f.

Elkins, G, A Johnson, and W Fisher. Cognitive hypnotherapy for pain management. *Am J Clin Hypn.* 2012 Apr;54(4):294–310.

Ertel, KA, MM Glymour, and LF Berkman. Effects of social integration on preserving memory function in a nationally representative US elderly population. *Am J Public Health*. 2008 Jul;98(7):1215–1220. Epub 2008 May 29.

Field, T. Tai chi research review. *Complement Ther Clin Pract*. 2011 Aug;17(3):141–146. Epub 2010 Oct 24.

Findlay, G. Abnormal brain activity in patients who cope poorly with back pain. *The Back Letter*. 2006 July;21(7):75.

Fishman, S, JC Ballantyne, and JP Rathmell. *Bonica's Management of Pain*, 4th Edition. Philadelphia: Lippincott Williams & Wilkins, 2010.

Friedly, J, L Chan, and R Deyo. Increases in lumbosacral injections in the Medicare population: 1994 to 2001. *Spine* (Phila Pa 1976). 2007 Jul 15;32(16):1754–1760.

Furlan, AD, L Brosseau, M Imamura, and E Irvin. Massage for low-back pain: a systematic review within the framework of the Cochrane Collaboration Back Review Group. *Spine* (Phila Pa 1976). 2002 Sep 1;27(17):1896–1910.

Goertz, CM, et al. Adding chiropractic manipulative therapy to standard medical care for patients with acute low back pain: results of a pragmatic randomized comparative effectiveness study. *Spine* (Phila Pa 1976). 2013 Apr 15;38(8):627–34. doi: 10.1097/BRS.0b013e31827733e7.

Golish, SR, et al. Outcome of lumbar epidural steroid injection is predicted by assay of a complex of fibronectin and aggrecan from epidural lavage. *Spine* (Phila Pa 1976). 2011 Aug 15;36(18):1464–1469.

Gujar, N, SS Yoo, P Hu, and MP Walker. Sleep deprivation amplifies reactivity of brain reward networks, biasing the appraisal of positive emotional experiences. *J Neurosci*. 2011 Mar 23;31(12): 4466–4474.

Gwilym, SE, N Filippini, G Douaud, AJ Carr, and I Tracey. Thalamic atrophy associated with painful osteoarthritis of the hip is reversible after arthroplasty: a longitudinal voxel-based morpho-metric study. *Arthritis Rheum.* 2010 Oct;62(10):2930–2940.

Haake, M, et al. German Acupuncture Trials (GERAC) for chronic low back pain: randomized, multicenter, blinded, parallel-group trial with 3 groups. *Arch Intern Med.* 2007 Sep 24;167(17):1892–1898.

Hoffman, BM, RK Papas, DK Chatkoff, and RD Kerns. Meta-analysis of psychological interventions for chronic low back pain. *Health Psychol.* 2007 Jan;26(1):1–9.

Hollinghurst, S, et al. Randomised controlled trial of Alexander technique lessons, exercise, and massage (ATEAM) for chronic and recurrent back pain: economic evaluation. *BMJ.* 2008 Dec 11; 337:a2656. doi: 10.1136/bmj.a2656

Jensen, MC, et al. Magnetic resonance imaging of the lumbar spine in people without back pain. *N Engl J Med.* 1994 Jul 14;331(2): 69–73.

Johnstone, T, CM van Reekum, HL Urry, NH Kalin, and RJ David-son. Failure to regulate: counterproductive recruitment of top-down prefrontal-subcortical circuitry in major depression. *J Neurosci.* 2007 Aug 15;27(33):8877–8884.

Jordan, KP, RA Hayward, M Blagojevic-Bucknall, and P Croft. In-cidence of prostate, breast, lung and colorectal cancer following new consultation for musculoskeletal pain: a cohort study among UK primary care patients. *Int J Cancer.* 2013 Aug 1;133(3):713–20. Epub 2013 Feb 25. doi: 10.1002/ijc.28055.

Kabir, SMR. Blog entry on Thursday, December 2, 2010, at the Spine Blog, From the desk of Syed M.R. Kabir, FRCSEd. http://journals.lww.com/spinejournal/blog/SpineBlog/pages/post.aspx?Post ID=37.

Kallmes, DF, et al. A randomized trial of vertebroplasty for osteopo-rotic spinal fractures. *N Engl J Med.* 2009 Aug 6;361(6):569–579.

Kell, RT, and GJ Asmundson. A comparison of two forms of periodized exercise rehabilitation programs in the management of chronic nonspecific low-back pain. *J Strength Cond Res.* 2009 Mar;23(2):513–523.

Kendall, NAS, SJ Linton, and C Main. Psychosocial Yellow Flags for acute low back pain: 'Yellow Flags'; as an analogue to 'Red Flags.' *European Journal of Pain.* 1998;(2):87–89. doi: 10.1016/S1090-3801 (98)90050-7.

Kruluwich, R, and J Abumrad. "How Do You Amputate A Phantom Limb?" *Morning Edition* of NPR; March 18, 2009. Accessed online at http://www.npr.org/templates/story/story.php?storyId=1017 88221 on September 15, 2012.

Lakadamyali, H, NC Tarhan, T Ergun, B Cakir, and AM Agildere. STIR sequence for depiction of degenerative changes in posterior stabilizing elements in patients with lower back pain. *AJR Am J Roentgenol.* 2008 Oct;191(4):973–979.

Landau, WM, DA Nelson, C Armon, CE Argoff, J Samuels, and MM Backonja. Assessment: use of epidural steroid injections to treat radicular lumbosacral pain: report of the Therapeutics and Technology Assessment Subcommittee of the American Academy of Neurology. *Neurology.* 2007 Aug 7;69(6):614; author reply 614–5.

Lee, MS, MII Pittler, and E Ernst. Internal qigong for pain conditions: a systematic review. *J Pain.* 2009 Nov;10(11):1121–1127.e14. Epub 2009 Jun 25.

Lehrer, J. The psychology of pain. *The Best Life.* 2008 Feb.

Liddle, SD, GD Baxter, and JH Gracey. Exercise and chronic low back pain: what works? *Pain.* 2004 Jan;107(1-2):176-90.

Little, P. Randomised controlled trial of Alexander technique lessons, exercise, and massage (ATEAM) for chronic and recurrent back pain. *BMJ.* 2008 Aug 19;337:a884. doi: 10.1136/bmj.a884.

Luijsterburg, PA, AP Verhagen, RW Ostelo, TA van Os, WC Peul, and BW Koes. Effectiveness of conservative treatments for the lumbosacral radicular syndrome: a systematic review. *Eur Spine J.* 2007 Jul;16(7):881–899. Epub 2007 Apr 6.

Luijsterburg, PA, et al. Cost-effectiveness of physical therapy and general practitioner care for sciatica. *Spine* (Phila Pa 1976). 2007 Aug 15;32(18):1942–1948.

Melzack, R, and PD Wall. Pain mechanisms: a new theory. *Science*. 1965 Nov 19;150(3699):971–979.

Millecamps, M. D-cycloserine reduces neuropathic pain behavior through limbic NMDA-mediated circuitry. *Pain*. 2007 Nov;132 (1-2):108–23. Epub 2007 Apr 20.

Mooney, V, and J Robertson. The facet syndrome. *Clin Orthop Relat Res*. 1976 Mar–Apr;(115):149–56.

Morone, NE, CM Greco, and DK Weiner. Mindfulness meditation for the treatment of chronic low back pain in older adults: a randomized controlled pilot study. *Pain*. 2008 Feb;134(3):310–319. Epub 2007 Jun 1.

Nerurkar, A, G Yeh, RB Davis, G Birdee, and RS Phillips. When conventional medical providers recommend unconventional medicine: results of a national study. *Arch Intern Med*. 2011 May 9;171(9): 862–864.

Nguyen, TH, DC Randolph, J Talmage, P Succop, and R Travis. Long-term outcomes of lumbar fusion among workers' compensation subjects: a historical cohort study. *Spine* (Phila Pa 1976). 2011 Feb 15;36(4):320–331.

Nielson, WR, and R Weir. Biopsychosocial approaches to the treatment of chronic pain. *Clin J Pain*. 2001 Dec;17(4 Suppl):S114–127.

O'Sullivan, RL, G Lipper, and EA Lerner. The neuro-immuno-cutaneous-endocrine network: relationship of mind and skin. *Arch Dermatol*. 1998 Nov;134(11):1431–435.

Parker-Pope, T. What are friends for? A longer life. *New York Times*, April 20, 2009.

Patel, AA, WR Spiker, M Daubs, D Brodke, and LA Cannon-Albright. Evidence for an inherited predisposition to lumbar disc disease. *J Bone Joint Surg Am*. 2011 Feb 2;93(3):225–229.

Patel, S, T Friede, R Froud, DW Evans, and M Underwood. Systematic review of randomised controlled trials of clinical prediction rules for physical therapy in low back pain. *Spine* (Phila Pa 1976). 2012 Dec 11.

Pearson, A. Blog entry on Thursday, December 2, 2010, at the Spine Blog, Interspinous devices: when will we know if they work? http://journals.lww.com/spinejournal/blog/SpineBlog/pages/post.aspx?PostID=38.

Pearson, AM, et al. Who should have surgery for degenerative spondylolisthesis? Treatment effect predictors in SPORT. *Spine* (Phila Pa 1976). 2013 Jul 10.

Peul WC, et al. Surgery versus prolonged conservative treatment for sciatica. *N Engl J Med.* 2007 May 31;356(22):2245-2256.

Price, L. Bent spines. *New York Times*, February 25, 2011. Available online at http://www.nytimes.com/2011/02/27/books/review/Price-t.html?pagewanted=all&_.

Rainville, J, R Nguyen, and P Suri. Effective conservative treatment for chronic low back pain. *Semin Spine Surg.* 2009 Dec 1;21(4): 257–263.

Ramachandran, VS, and D Brang. Sensations evoked in patients with amputation from watching an individual whose corresponding intact limb is being touched. *Arch Neurol.* 2009 Oct;66(10): 1281–1284

Raspe, H, A Hueppe, and H Neuhauser. Back pain, a communicable disease? *Int J Epidemiol.* 2008 Feb;37(1):69–74. Epub 2007 Nov 17.

Reichenbach, S, and JN Katz. Commentary: When East meets West—comments on "Back pain as a communicable disease." *Int J Epidemiol.* 2008 Feb;37(1):74–76. Epub 2008 Jan 31.

Rutkowski, MD, BA Winkelstein, WF Hickey, JL Pahl, and JA DeLeo. Lumbar nerve root injury induces central nervous system neuroimmune activation and neuroinflammation in the rat: relationship to painful radiculopathy. *Spine* (Phila Pa 1976). 2002 Aug 1;27(15):1604–1613.

Rutkowski, MD, and JA DeLeo. The role of cytokines in the initiation and maintenance of chronic pain. *Drug News Perspect.* 2002 Dec;15(10):626–632.

Saravanakumar, K. *Bonica's Management of Pain.* 4th ed. *Anaesthesia.* 2010 Jun 24. [Epub ahead of print].

Sarno, J. *Healing Back Pain: The Mind-Body Connection.* New York: Grand Central (reprint edition), 2010.

Sasaki, N, et al. Physical exercise affects cell proliferation in lumbar intervertebral disc regions in rats. *Spine* (Phila Pa 1976). 2012 Aug 1;37(17):1440–1447. doi: 10.1097/BRS.0b013e31824ff87d

Schwartz, DR, and CE Carney. Mediators of cognitive-behavioral therapy for insomnia: a review of randomized controlled trials and secondary analysis studies. *Clin Psychol Rev.* 2012 Nov;32(7): 664–675. Epub 2012 Jul 3.

Sembrano, JN, and DW Polly Jr. How often is low back pain not coming from the back? *Spine* (Phila Pa 1976). 2009 Jan 1;34(1):E27–32.

Simons, DG. Cardiology and myofascial trigger points: Janet G. Travell's contribution. *Tex Heart Inst J.* 2003;30(1):3–7.

Simons, DG, JG Travell, LS Simons, and BD Cummings. *Travell & Simons' Myofascial Pain and Dysfunction: The Trigger Point Manual.* 2nd ed. New York: Lippincott Williams & Wilkins, 1998.

Spengler, DM, et al. Back injuries in industry: a retrospective study. I. Overview and cost analysis. *Spine* (Phila Pa 1976). 1986 Apr;11(3): 241–245.

Strömqvist, BH, et al. X-stop versus decompressive surgery for lumbar neurogenic intermittent claudication: randomized controlled trial with 2-year follow-up. *Spine* (Phila Pa 1976). 2013 Aug 1;38(17): 1436–1442. doi: 10.1097/BRS.0b013e31828ba413

Sweitzer, SM, WF Hickey, MD Rutkowski, JL Pahl, and JA DeLeo. Focal peripheral nerve injury induces leukocyte trafficking into the central nervous system: potential relationship to neuropathic pain. *Pain.* 2002 Nov;100(1-2):163–170.

Szczurko, O, et al. Naturopathic care for chronic low back pain: a randomized trial. *PLoS One.* 2007 Sep 19;2(9):e919.

Tomé-Bermejo, F, A Barriga-Martín, and JL Martín. Identifying patients with chronic low back pain likely to benefit from lumbar facet radiofrequency denervation: a prospective study. *J Spinal Disord Tech*. 2011 Apr;24(2):69–75.

Tsao, H, LA Danneels, and PW Hodges. ISSLS prize winner: Smudging the motor brain in young adults with recurrent low back pain. *Spine* (Phila Pa 1976). 2011 Oct 1;36(21):1721–1727.

Tsao, JC. Effectiveness of massage therapy for chronic, non-malignant pain: a review. *Evid Based Complement Alternat Med*. 2007 Jun;4(2):165–79. Epub 2007 Feb 5.

Vann, M. Biofeedback for back pain. Accessed online at http://www .everydayhealth.com. on September 14, 2012.

Walker, MP, and E van der Helm. Overnight therapy? The role of sleep in emotional brain processing. *Psychol Bull*. 2009 Sep;135(5): 731–748.

Watanabe, K, et al. Clinical outcomes of posterior lumbar interbody fusion for lumbar foraminal stenosis: preoperative diagnosis and surgical strategy. *J Spinal Disord Tech*. 2011 May;24(3):137–141.

Wechsler, A. *The Mind-Beauty Connection: 9 Days to Less Stress, Gorgeous Skin, and a Whole New You*. New York: Free Press, 2009.

Weinstein, JA, et al. Surgical versus nonoperative treatment for lumbar disc herniation: four-year results for the Spine Patient Outcomes Research Trial (SPORT). *Spine* (Phila Pa 1976). 2008 Dec 1;33(25):2789–2800.

Weinstein, JN. Balancing science and informed choice in decisions about vertebroplasty. *N Engl J Med*. 2009 Aug 6;361(6):619–621.

Weinstein, JN, et al. Surgical versus nonsurgical treatment for lumbar degenerative spondylolisthesis. *N Engl J Med*. 2007 May 31;356(22): 2257–2270.

Weistroffer, JK, and WK Hsu. Return-to-play rates in National Football League linemen after treatment for lumbar disk herniation. *Am J Sports Med*. 2011 Mar;39(3):632–636. Epub 2011 Jan 10.

Willems, PC, JB Staal, GH Walenkamp, and RA de Bie. Spinal fusion for chronic low back pain: systematic review on the accuracy of tests for patient selection. *Spine J.* 2013 Feb;13(2):99–109. doi: 10.1016/j.spinee.2012.10.001. Epub 2012 Nov 3.

Yoo, SS, N Gujar, P Hu, FA Jolesz, and MP Walker. The human emotional brain without sleep—a prefrontal amygdala disconnect. *Curr Biol.* 2007 Oct 23;17(20):R877–878.

Online Resources

- The Association for Applied Psychophysiology and Biofeedback, Inc.: www.aapb.org
- National Association of Cognitive-Behavioral Therapists: www.nacbt.org
- American Hypnosis Association: www.hypnosis.edu
- American Psychological Association: www.apa.org
- Center for Mental Health Services Knowledge Exchange Network: www.mentalhealth.org
- The Center for Mindfulness at the University of Massachusetts Medical School: www.umassmed.edu/cfm/home
- The American Physical Therapy Association: www.moveforward pt.com
- The American Society for the Alexander Technique: www.amsat online.org
- The Biofeedback Certification International Alliance: www.bcia .org
- The Qi Gong Institute: www.qigonginstitute.org
- Sleep Foundation: www.sleepfoundation.org

Index

action plans
    failed back syndrome, 144–45
    history and analysis of pain, 23
    integrative therapies, 184
    lifestyle interventions, 263
    partnership with doctor, 72–73
    psychological issues, 199–201, 222–23
    treatment protocols, 91
    understanding pain generators, 48–49
acupuncture, 151–52, 165–68
adjacent segment disease, 142, 144
aerobic exercise, 179, 239–42
Alexander Technique, 168–69, 218
alternative therapies. *See* integrative
    therapies
anti-inflammatory diet, 261–62
anti-inflammatory drugs, 38, 83, 96, 161
Apkarian, A. Vania, 192
Armon, Carmel, 162
arthritis
    anti-inflammatory diet for, 260
    brain shrinkage from, 195
    collagen vascular disease, 62, 122
    from disc dehydration, 45
    exercise therapies, 157, 168, 179
    facet joint problems, 83, 115, 132
    neural foramen pain, 49
    osteophytes (bone spurs), 85, 95, 101
arthrodesis (spinal fusion), 20–21, 97, 103–4,
    139, 144
artificial disc replacement, 97
attitudes. *See* psychological factors
axial pain generators
    bones, 36–38
    muscles, 31–33
    soft tissues, 33–36

back biomechanics, 28–29
back pain. *See also* pain generators
    action plan, 23
    books and scientific papers about, 274–84
    characteristics and history, 3–7, 63–64,
        268, 269
    cultural factors, 12–16
    five-step treatment program, xxi–xxiii,
        265–71
    lifetime risk and rate of recurrence, 9–10
    multiplicity of causes and factors, 10–11,
        69, 79
    online resources for information, 285
    online tools and updates, www
        .drjackstern.com, xxv, 4, 63, 271, 274
    types and categories, 11–12, 38, 196
Baliki, Marwan N., 192–93
beliefs. *See* psychological factors
biofeedback, 175–76, 209, 215–17
biomechanics of back function, 28–29
bones
    benign tumors, 127
    cancer, 37, 127–28, 137–38
    cancer detection, 82, 88, 123–24
    cancer-related fractures, 123
    osteoporotic compression fractures, 37, 82,
        121–27
    as pain generators, 36–37, 121
    spondylolysis and spondylolisthesis,
        129–34
    spurs (osteophytes), 85, 95, 101
    stress fractures, 129–34
    trauma, 128–29, 134
brain. *See* psychological factors;
        psychological interventions and
        mind-body techniques